D1312973

Seeds
of
Mindfulness

SEEDS

of

MINDFULNESS

101

Mindful Moments in the Garden

Fiann Ó Nualláin

ixia
PRESS

Garden City, New York

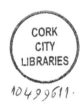

Copyright

Bibliographical Note

Seeds of Mindfulness: 101 Mindful Moments in the Garden is a new work, first published by Ixia Press in 2021.

Library of Congress Cataloging-in-Publication Data

Names: Ó Nualláin, Fiann, author.
Title: Seeds of mindfulness : 101 mindful moments in the garden / Fiann Ó Nualláin.
Description: Garden City, New York : IXIA Press, [2021] | Includes bibliographical references. | Summary: "To mindfully garden is both deeply enrichingand easy to achieve. This delightful compilation offers more than 100 mindful gardening moments that combine a spiritual practice with a favorite pastime"—Provided by publisher.
Identifiers: LCCN 2020023074 | ISBN 9780486845388 (trade paperback)
Subjects: LCSH: Gardening—Therapeutic use. | Mindfulness (Psychology)
Classification: LCC RM735.7.G37 O583 2021 | DDC 615.8/515—dc23
LC record available at https://lccn.loc.gov/2020023074

IXIA PRESS
An imprint of Dover Publications, Inc.

Manufactured in the United States by LSC Communications
84538901
www.doverpublications.com/ixiapress

2 4 6 8 10 9 7 5 3 1

2020

For green thumbs and verdant hearts

Preface

"If you wish to make anything grow, you must understand it, and understand it in a very real sense. 'Green fingers' are a fact, and a mystery only to the unpracticed. But green fingers are the extensions of a verdant heart."

—Montague Russell Page

I am a lifelong gardener; it is sort of in my DNA—with both my grandfathers of green fingers and both my grandmothers of verdant hearts. My dad was a keen gardener, too, so apart from raking and watering being on my chore list, I learned at his side to appreciate nature and grow with it. Over the years, I found such solace and inspiration in the garden that I eventually took it up as a profession as well as a passion. I initially trained in horticulture and crop science but soon found a fascination with medicinal botany and horticultural therapy.

I have worked for two decades as a horticultural therapist, and in that role, I encourage people—be they lifelong gardeners, novices, or the never ventured—to find health, well-being, resilience, and mindfulness through the garden and the practice of gardening. I encourage them to embrace the garden as a therapeutic space and take on the therapy benefits of the pastime—to pass the time in a manner more productive to the self than being caught up in thoughts, stresses, or diagnosis.

The "time-out" in the garden is psychologically—and spiritually—beneficial, and many of the physical tasks are conducive not just to occupational therapy but also delivering better brain chemistry toward positive mood and stronger well-being perception. I trained in a wide protocol of psychological supports, including psychotherapy, cognitive behavioral therapy, addiction studies, stress reduction techniques, mindfulness facilitation, and holistic therapies. What I learned was easy to incorporate into the garden because much of it grows there naturally.

Gardening offers the opportunity to experience awe, wonder, and peak experience as well as satisfaction, happiness, contentment, achievement, self-fulfillment, self-awareness, and a grounded self. It promotes optimism and gratitude toward its rewards. It gifts positive regard for nature and enthusiasm toward connection to the natural world. There is noticing, loving-kindness, and nonstriving all present right there in that connection. We automatically relax in a garden and become more physically and mentally receptive to a mindful, restorative, or healing experience.

In this book, calling upon my lifelong personal experience and my professional insights, I explore gardening moments and motivations that support those mindful, restorative, and healing experiences. I gather the healthiest and most attractive seeds of gardening therapy and mindful practices—ones with a good track record, ones with no fuss, and ones easy to germinate and selected to thrive. Ones to delight the heart and open the mind. Ones to empty the mind and fill the soul.

Introduction

Mindfulness Is . . .

Mindfulness is the achievement of an "awake presence"—to be fully realized and cognizant in the moment or at any given moment, what some call "being in the now." It is a focused self, fully aware and participating in the moment, in what is happening, in the life of your own being—not sleepwalking or daydreaming through the moment, circumstance, or situation. It is you being here—right here, right now, awake and present.

As a spiritual tool—best known in the Buddhist tradition and a key practice on the path to enlightenment—entering into the "attentive awareness" of mindfulness is a way of switching your spirit on, of manifesting your pure reality. In this space, your alive essence is unhindered by ego and emotions, and the you without layers of conditioning—one might even say "the natural you"—emerges.

In this more natural state, where the reality of things is not clouded by thought biases or emotionally triggered judgments or preconceptions, your psychological self actually experiences the world or a situation—and your part in it—for what it really is. You could say it is the real you in real time living a real life.

As a psychological tool, mindfulness meditation and mindful practices are seen as a way to liberate yourself from the clutter of dissonant thoughts and manage the pings, pangs, and stings of life's vicissitudes. It is not just attaining a peace of mind but also attaining neuroplasticity—retraining how the signaling brain reacts, bringing more self-control. Being in the now—right here, right now, awake and present—there is neither time nor place for catastrophizing or becoming overwhelmed.

Mindfulness has a role in day-to-day stress reduction, in caring for your mental health, and in improving your quality of life—to be mindful (focused) is not to be mindfull (thought-cluttered). It is not emptying of all thoughts; it is not denial or avoidance. It is that you are considerate of what thoughts are arising or moving through, and you can acknowledge the thought and even its emotion but not grasp at it; simply let it keep going without disrupting your spirit or your time. It is a most productive therapy, as every thought let go is one you're not fixing your mindset to. You can adapt yourself to respond rather than react. There is choice in the situation; there is a means of control.

Mindfulness is a means of how we experience the reality of the now. That now is not always a static meditation or in a therapeutic setting. It may be on the busy commute when you take a moment to follow your breath or appreciate the view from the window. It may be making the bed, mowing the lawn, or even reading a book with your full self switched on. It is how you experience what you are doing. You can mindfully walk the dog, mindfully wash the car, or mindfully eat a meal. Anything can be done in mindful mode—except panic.

Yes, there may be trepidation on the first few steps of any new or renewed venture, but there is no need to panic. Being mindful is simply being aware of what it is you are doing while you are doing it. That's it. From that, other things spring and bear fruit. It is not attempting to achieve a state of perpetual grace—a permanent state of being fully present; occasional daydreams and zoning out are good for the psychological self too. But it is not so elusive either. You can enter it at will—after a little practice—and over time, the mindfulness increases and even occurs without willpower required. It can become, with time, your default setting.

For now, you can switch it on with intent, you can switch it on by using your senses and your focus, you can follow your breath or use a mantra or trigger, and you can and will switch it on with the moments and motivations in this book. It is not across the room; it is here, now. It may be at the end of the garden, but it is here and now too. Get it where and when you can. Get it by doing more of it. Get it by "being" more in it.

A Twofold Path

There are two ways to achieve mindfulness—one is in stillness, and the other is in action. The garden gifts both; it is full of actions to be taken in a mindful way, and it presents plenty of opportunities for stillness and meditative modes too.

The still mode is a mindful or attentive meditation, generally achieved by following and focusing on your breath—in and out, in and out—and returning to the deliberate attention of the inhale and exhale whenever you notice that you have wandered off the path into thoughts. It can also be achieved with a mantra. The focus on the breath or mantra is the removal of all other distractions—it is the focused, alert, and fully present self in that moment and into the next, as long as the meditation lasts.

This moment-to-moment attunement wires the brain for fuller concentration capacity and fuller (if not also higher) consciousness—not just within the meditation but also in the rest of your life. You can use the breath method as your daily mindful meditation or as the "on" button for entering mindful phases throughout the day.

Stillness doesn't have to be all about following the breath or sitting in a meditative posture. You can be equally engaged in mindfulness by a sensory awareness during a moment out or even in the middle of a task. Something like feeling the sun on your face as you mow the lawn or plant in the border is also an opportunity to find that mindful moment—to make that moment mindful. You can hone in on the sun experience, absorbing its warmth, expressing gratitude, or acknowledging the pleasure or pleasant feeling it stirs. You are not ignoring the thoughts or feelings; you are engaged with them in an alert manner. You are paying attention to the positivity of the moment. It is the "being in it" that is the "awake presence" of mindfulness practice.

There is great potential in honing in on a sense experience and letting go of it—releasing yourself to the goodness of the sensation and experience. You can if you choose to follow your breath in the moment. You can drink it all in and even make a smile or positive noises—that's just marking it. It's a moment—have it. It is doing you good; acknowledge it. When you are done, you can return to finish the task you started—or back to sitting still or a specific breath exercise or recited mantra.

A lot of the emphasis on mindfulness by modern mindful practitioners, and back to early Buddhist texts, is about the letting go, the emptying, the nonclinging to thoughts and emotions—and, yes, it is that: to be liberated from attachment to a reactionary brain. But with mindfulness comes *sampajanna*, or clear comprehension, and not all thoughts and emotions need to be dismissed; some are worth experiencing mindfully. Mindfulness provides the discernment to pick and choose what we bring into our now and what we let pass on by.

The action mode is just as simple. You will not need a stunt double—just a mindful approach or a switched-on self in the performance of a task. It is "being" in the "doing." It can happen in any aspect of your everyday life. Eating your lunch, washing the laundry, and mowing the lawn all can be done not just with alertness but with presence of self— mindfully.

Simply follow your breath into the now, and allow yourself to be fully there in the task without thoughts or judgments. Let your senses guide you—be with them. When you eat next, be fully awake to the flavor in your chew. When you do laundry next, experience the sights, sounds, and textures around you.

When you mow next, don't just walk; actually feel the ground beneath your feet while you're in motion.

Bringing your attention to the task or action transforms it into a mindful exercise. Soon those exercises teach the brain—and, we might say, the mind-body-spirit—to switch on the mindful mode more and more automatically. Then in the more aware state of experience—in and of the action—we can appreciate it fully, be respectful and receiving of it, and experience gratitude or loving-compassion within it.

Mindfulness is heightened experience; mindfulness is true self without the distraction of thinking or wandering into thoughts that diminish the experience. It is being present for what's going on as it is going on. This is a life not daydreamed or sleepwalked through. This is a life lived.

At first you may have to adhere to some regimented practice—breath exercises and catching the drift—to acquire the skill of mindful focus, but then you can be more fluid with it. So while at first, mindfully washing laundry means doing the chore with a moment or two of mindfulness activation to it (during it), soon it will be an opportunity to be mindfully activated for the entirety of the task. You will be alert for the whole task—the doing of it or *in the flow* of it—and not randomly thinking about what you're going to make for dinner. Think Zen monks raking a gravel garden—a task but also a prayer or a resilience exercise.

Following your breath as you mow or rake and being in the action of mowing or raking—and not thinking about the watering or weeding that comes next—is a mindful action;

that is an action meditation. The mowing or raking type of meditation is often the recommended entry point for making your gardening more mindful. It is a regular task reframed as a meditative moment, so it sets up the new mindset and makes all the other opportunities of mindful activation ripen into pleasant rewards.

Mindfulness is dynamic; you can shake it up. Maybe when you mow next, it's not about grounding yourself in the action or the solidity of the earth beneath your feet but rather the smell of the cut grass that wafts up into your nostrils. The breath following now is an inhale of a scent—pleasant to some, not so much to others—but judgment aside, that scent is the consequence and reality of your mowing. Experiencing it is the reality of what is going on. Acknowledging it is being in the now of mowing. That is coming to your senses to achieve mindfulness.

Mindful Gardening Is . . .

Mindful gardening is simply gardening with an "awake presence." It is being in the moment for the task or the lived moment with focus, with gratitude, with appreciation, with loving-compassion, with truth, with awareness, with a connection to the moment as it unfolds—with yourself. It is being there.

It may unfold in the "lost in the garden" experience, where self-consciousness and ego disappear. A pure oneness with nature and your role in it removes intrusive thoughts and enables an *in the flow* experience—that, too, is a liberated self—a peak experience mindfulness.

INTRODUCTION

The garden is a contemplative space and suited to hosting a mindful meditation—to be still and present in the moment—but it is also a place to find your senses and enter the now. To touch a textured plant, to taste an edible berry, to smell a fragrant shrub—all are portals to becoming aware of the experience, aware of this moment in your life, and aware of your living self.

Gardeners are vigilant to the water needs of the plants in their care and to pests and problems. The vigilant brain does not have to be on stress mode—it can be a managed attunement or a trained perceptiveness. When it comes to rewiring the brain, here is the automatic switch to "present focus" that gardening gifts.

Gardening is a moving meditation too—an action meditation. All of its tasks—watering, deadheading, planting, and weeding—are perfect opportunities for present moment awareness. It doesn't have to be a Zen garden to deliver a Zen experience. More and more people are practicing mindfulness in relation to a garden. In a way, you don't even need to follow your breath, just your passion.

So go garden. Go be mindful in your garden. Go be a more grounded and full potential self. Go. Be.

The Seeds

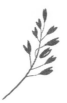

"All the flowers of all the tomorrows
are in the seeds of today."

—Indian proverb

To Make a Start

To make a start, one must start—it's that simple. You can plan for this and train for that and bide your time for the right moment, and all the while, the time is now. Now is the now of it. There is an apt Indian proverb that states, "All the flowers of all the tomorrows are in the seeds of today." Universally, we cannot all put off until tomorrow what we can do today.

You have opened the seed packet; that's a start—but sow them. Starts are a beginning—the next thing is ongoing. The now of mindfulness is not a single moment of awareness/peace/grace/enlightenment; it is the moment-to-moment living in a more attuned awareness/peace/grace/enlightenment. The gardener knows that opening the seed packet is only the start of the start. The sowing and watering and tending to until established—that's the deed to be done; that's the flourishing of the intent to sow.

Good starts are great, but following through is the real deal. Apply yourself, apply, apply—do. Apply, apply—become. If you truly seek mindfulness, then be mindful. Start now.

A First Seed to Sow

Following your breath is a key tenet of mindfulness. It is the seed that germinates to a bountiful experience.

Simply close your eyes for a moment, and quietly focus on your natural breathing pattern—hear it; feel it. Notice the inhale and how your body moves to it; notice the exhale and how your body reacts to it. It may be shallow and nasal now, or it may be deep and lung-filling; that's not the important part—not yet. Just notice it. Try to pay attention to it for twenty seconds—the in, the out, the in, the out. Any thoughts that come, let them come and go, and keep returning your focus to your breathing rhythm.

That's it. Job done. You have begun the journey. Mindfulness is that simple—returning your focus to the task at hand. In this instance, and in many ways, the concept of simply following your breath is the key that opens the mindful door. Breathing is your automatic life support system—this is you alive. Tuning in to it is tapping into the very engine of your existence. It is such a little thing to do, but it has such a powerful effect.

Later you can learn how to alter breathing patterns to strengthen the meditation, improve clarity of consciousness, and bolster health. But for now, following your breath for a few moments is the best starting point for this journey. The seed is sown; it will germinate with nurture. This seed does not need water; it needs oxygen and CO_2—the next mindful inhale, the next mindful exhale. Go!

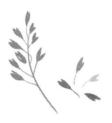

Seed Selection

We can think of our emotions and intentions as seeds. Those that we water will thrive; those that we don't give attention to will stay dormant or wither to nothing. So it is important to select the seeds we wish to cultivate and put our attention there.

Yes, we have within ourselves the seeds of anger, contempt, reticence, and self-doubt as well as the seeds of love, compassion, conservation, and joy. What are you growing now? What do you wish to grow?

This is your life; you can put the energy of it into what you want to see flourish. Thriving plants bulk up and, in doing so, leave less room for weeds. Sure, weeding will be required, but why not have a robust garden that can out-flourish the weeds. So be honest with yourself, and make the better choices. What are you growing now, and what do you wish to grow?

Task Selection

We can seek a harvest from mindfulness—the crop will be those seeds we sow: compassion, loving-kindness, resilience, spiritual fortitude, peace of mind, stress relief, and clarity.

It is not that we just wish for these seeds to germinate; we do not just scatter hope to the wind. We prepare a seed bed, sow it, and pay attention to it—nurture it. We nurture it by vigilant returns, checking back in with our compassion, loving-kindness, peace of mind, etc. We will tend and attend to our growing self. We will garden our being. That's the task. That's the undertaking—that's the great reward.

Mindfulness is not just a psychological state. To thrive, it must be incorporated into our whole self: into our physical world—into what we do and how we do. So to be a more mindful gardener, we can make a "to-do" or "to-be" list. We can stick it on the shed wall, and every time we go in for a tool, we can come out with a purpose— to prune with compassion, dig with resilience, mow with peace of mind, and rake with clarity.

"*The quality of your life depends on the seeds you water.
If you plant tomato seeds in your gardens,
tomatoes will grow. Just so, if you water a
seed of peace in your mind, peace will grow.*"

—Thich Nhat Hanh

Pacing Yourself

Mindful moments can be slowdown moments—taking the time to smell a flower or look at the sky, to sit on a bench and breathe, or to lie on a lawn and be present to the universe around and within you. Many people take to it as a relaxation technique. Fair enough, but mindfulness is really about being present, and that includes being present to all the gears of your day. You could mindfully sprint across the line, as most athletes are mindful in their winning moment—as well as in their training and other performances. They may call it focus, dedication, or the will to win, but they are at one with that purpose. They are all there. It is not just giving all; it is being your all in the now of the race.

There is no starter gun in the garden; there is no finish line either. But we do exert our physicality, and so we can and should be mindful in the doing too—in the moments where we have to pick up the pace as well as the peaceful interludes. If we are present in the chore, it is no longer a chore; it is a mindful exercise. The garden has plenty of opportunities to slow or pick up the pace.

Don't feel you have to be in mindful mode 24/7. You don't even have to be trying to make every chore mindful; the garden will present opportunities, and you can create opportunities. You can choose just to water today and even daydream through it—it's your life; take it at your pace. This way you won't force doing; you will be you as you do. That's the tao of it—that's the flowering of mindfulness.

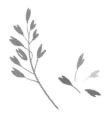

Gardening Tasks

Becoming a more mindful gardener does not pit "being" over "doing." To garden is to do—how we do is also how we be. We can carry out our daily chores as mindful practices. We can rake like a Zen monk for sure, but we can also mow the lawn with attention—be there as we do it.

Often, the monotonous tasks of life are done on autopilot, but if we are present in the moment, they are not so monotonous. We are alive in the moment of their doing—the doing is a vibrational lift to our being when it is done mindfully.

Being present is experiencing life. Being present is the root of mindful gardening. Doing what needs to be done in the garden today with focus and conscious presence is mindful gardening. You may have been doing it all along but didn't notice. Mindfulness will sharpen your noticing. To notice is mindfulness. In noticing, the doing of the task is the witnessing of the now of it and brings our being into the task. We are truly there—that is the aim and actualizing of mindfulness.

To Sow Mindfully

Sowing seed is not an act of will. It is participation in the divine force of creation; it is participation in the force of life—to renew itself. In sowing seed, you are present at the conception of a new batch of plants. Be present. Be awestruck. Be joyous. Be mindful.

With diligence, read the seed packet or recall from past experience the seed's requirements to germinate. Does it need light, so a surface sowing? Does it germinate in darkness, so a prod of a pencil tip to set its depth in the growing media? This attention to detail is being present to the life process requirements of the plant. Taking it seriously—not just dispersing seed any old way and leaving it to chance—is not just due diligence but rather respect. Respect is loving-kindness—it is an open heart; it is an awake presence to the undertaking.

Bring your awake presence to every stage—to filling the compost tray or making the drill or fine tilth in the earth. Put or manifest the intent for success in every action. Feel the seed in your hand, and carefully deposit it into its position to grow. Consciously water it to its required needs. This may be a gardening task that you do regularly, almost on muscle memory, without experiencing. But why not experience it anew by doing it as if for the first time, by letting it be the full focus of your attention? By being here and now with it.

To Plant Mindfully

I n the section on sowing a seed mindfully, I mentioned diligence. Diligence is acting with integrity; it is bringing your dutiful and alert self into the process. We gardeners can become automatic with regular gardening tasks and not really be present to what we are doing. We may dig a hole with the right depth and water in after planting, but perhaps we "phone it in" or go through the motions without actually noticing what we are doing or have done. To plant mindfully is not just to bring a correct method to bear; it is to be there.

So notice how you dig the hole; feel the implement in your hand or how your hand parts the soil. Feel it; register it. Become aware of the plant as you tip it from its pot, tease it roots, and place it in the hole. Feel the sensation of backfilling, firming in—there is a lot of physicality and contact here. Experience it all. Then with positive regard, water the plant. Know that you have given it the best start you can. Know that by planting with your attentive self, in a mindful mode, you have really interacted with that plant—that you have cultivated a connection, that you are not just *doing* in the garden, that you are *being* and a vital part of *its* being.

"Where would the gardener be if there were no more weeds?"

—Zhuang Zhou

To Weed Mindfully

Like any good gardening book or visit to a garden, there will be plenty of prompts to get weeding across these pages—often alluding to the spiritual and psychological significance of weeding negativity from your life in order to allow space for positivity to grow. Weeding is a great metaphor, but we are gardeners and gardens have actual weeds, so some actual weeding will be done.

We can weed a physical weed mindfully and bring our attention to how it may resist or give way to our pulling hand. We are not relishing its destruction; rather, we are acknowledging that it has to go—that it competes for water, nutrients, space, and even light. It may seem that we are being judgmental; we are not. We are simply acknowledging, accepting, and responding accordingly. Many gardeners root out a bramble or nettle with judgmental attitude, with curses and even aggression, but why waste all that energy? Why manifest contempt? We weed for the greater good of the garden, so do it in the spirit of goodness.

We can be present to the weeds' removal—actually witness it. We may notice how the hoe or other tool is efficient. We may reflect some gratitude for such inventions and the easing of our labor. I like to think of weeding as harvesting material for the compost heap. Any negative associations—as well as the monotony of a mundane chore—are thus transformed into a purposeful action that can be carried out as a dynamic mindful exercise. Of course, some days it's just weeding, and that's okay— but the more we do it mindfully, the more mindful we become.

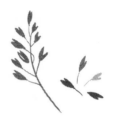

Awake Presence

Mindfulness can be seen as your "awake presence." It is awareness and presence in the now of what you are experiencing. It is being awake and present to your life in all or any of its being and doing. It is what you can bring to the moment; it is what brings you alive in the moment. Some consider it a heightened self; I see it as a truer self. It is a more dynamic self because when you are awake and present, you truly get to experience the moment: to feel the real, to be real. Yes, it is a cognition boost; yes, it is a performance boost. But it's also a focus of your life force.

Your awake presence is your full potential not goaded by societal conditioning or any external complications. This is a purer you. Are you awake? Are you present? Don't sleepwalk or daydream through life—live it. Are you awake? Are you present? Really now, be real in this now. Are you awake? Are you present?

Ask yourself whenever you need to. Ask yourself if that sparks the moment. Ask, ask, hear. Awake, awaken your presence, be of the now right now. Yes, awake. Yes, present.

To Mindfully Attune

Conscious awareness is the aim and attainment of mindfulness. It is both a practiced skill and a living state. It is how you enter the now and what entering the now gifts.

To mindfully attune is to focus the mind to clarity—to not be caught up in rumination or thought-surfing. It is simply to be your unhindered self, present in the moment, present to each moment, moment by moment. It is being awake or alert to reality, being there, being here right now. It is being in the now.

It can be called awareness, and it is often called enlightenment. But it is not a thing to achieve—a one-off transformation. It is more like the transforming dynamic. You do not take a single breath and live; you keep breathing and living simultaneously—that is the moment-to-moment of mindfulness.

To mindfully attune, you can follow your breath, you can experience one of your senses, you can meditate, you can close your eyes and radiate your inner being, and you can open your eyes and greet the world. You can even step out into the garden and be "gardener." The secret is to do what you are doing—to be who you are.

The Way to Be Can Be to Do

Lao Tzu, the Chinese Taoist philosopher (circa the fifth or sixth century BCE), is believed to have decreed, "The way to do is to be." In addition, the way to be can be to do.

It is no wonder that both contemplative Christian monks and Zen Buddhist monks took up gardening as part of their spiritual life—the grounding and commitment of maintaining an herb garden and the discipline and patience of raking a gravel path. These dedications are devotion. These tasks are prayer.

This doing opens the self to being—whether that's closer to God or closer to no-mind doesn't really matter. It's the being right there that is the transformative or enlightening power. Whatever your next gardening task, do it mindfully and deepen your awareness to its transformative power. You don't need the robes or the haircut, but you can say "om" or "amen."

"Nature does not hurry yet everything is accomplished."

—Lao Tzu

In Tune with Our Circadian Rhythm

Just as plants react to daylight, soil moisture, or ambient temperature, so, too, we humans take similar cues from the natural world. In us, daylight triggers the activation of an alert neurotransmitter called serotonin, which wakes us up to be active in daytime, while lowlight or nighttime prompts the release of a sedating hormone—melatonin—to make us sleepy and go rest up. This is known as the circadian rhythm.

One of the stress factors of the modern world is that working or living under artificial light during daylight actually triggers melatonin, and looking at phones and screens in the evening triggers serotonin—so our rhythms are offbeat. No wonder we are tired all the time. The answer is to get outside.

Being and doing in the garden in the bright of day is you truly experiencing the day—the reality of it and the purposeful serotonin release of it. You are truly operating on a daytime setting. If you have to be at work all day and only get to garden in the evening, then being and doing in the garden in the ebbing light of the evening is you truly experiencing the transition of day toward night—and in the reality of it, this is the purposeful prompt to melatonin levels and a shift in brain waves toward a better night's sleep, which will improve your daytime energy tomorrow.

It doesn't matter when you tend the garden; it tends you back.

Cultivating Neuroplasticity

L eisure swimmers have different muscles compared to committed cyclists, and gardening works muscles that typing won't. Just as muscles may be built by occupation, pastime, or determination, so, too, our brains are built upon by how they get worked—by experience, repeat experience, and ongoing flexing. It is not just that we can alter our attitudes. We can actually change our minds— physically rewire the structure of our brain by regularly adopting and flexing that attitude. The brain is pliable enough to change, to alter—it is not rigid; it has plasticity. Previous embedded mindsets can be unset.

Neuroplasticity is happening all the time. It is how we learn new things. What is interesting is that one must be up for it—enthusiasm is required. You can't really go through the motions of it—positive motivation and real alertness trigger the neurochemicals necessary to enable brain modifications. So your depressed state or distracted anxiousness actually switches your neuroplasticity function off. Coming to mindfulness is the way to reengage that function and activate purpose.

In learning any new task, the more honed the attention, the more you take it in and the more memory is retained for how to do so. It's the old "practice makes perfect" idiom; the more repetition, the more the brain grabs of the experience and the more it gets wired in. Each time, the brain strengthens the connections of neurons that are engaged in the task or experience. Cell-to-cell cooperation is enhanced in the moment-to-moment of the occurrence. When we bring moment-to-moment mindfulness to this process, we enhance it by reducing the disruptive power of distraction. We are there; it is happening—game on, switch on.

The single task of bringing our presence to the moment—to the task at hand—consolidates performance and perfects acquisition. The more you practice mindfulness, the more you cultivate your own neuroplasticity.

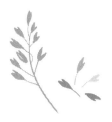

The Tao of Brain Restructuring

The way to rewire your brain is through flexing the right muscles or, more to the point, firing the right neurons and stimulating the right pathways. This is achieved by mindful meditations and incorporating more mindful approaches into daily life. That is the way, but what actually happens?

Mindfulness induces measurable changes in the brain structure. Just like a muscle that's repeatedly worked gets some bulk, so, too, is cortical thickness improved in regions of the brain lit up by mindful meditations and practices. Repeat attentive mindfulness thickens the anterior cingulate cortex, which is responsible for self-regulatory processes and cognitive flexibility. This attentive strengthening strengthens attention capacity.

Mindfulness meditation and equanimity exercises thicken the prefrontal cortex, which is responsible for problem-solving and regulating emotions, allowing for greater expression of self-control, harmony, and insight application. Mindfulness also works out the hippocampus, which directs learning and memory, helping to embed the outcomes of these structural changes. We remember to be more attentive, and we learn how to be more compassionate, more grateful, more attuned, and more in the moment. In doing, we become; in becoming, we are truly being.

Not everything is increased. In fact, regular mindfulness decreases the amygdala: the fight-or-flight center—the reactionary part of our brain and personality. It's the part bulked up by anxiety and fear. It is not that you will become risk-averse; you will have less doubt and less knee-jerk reaction. The clear comprehension that arrives from mindfulness is seeing that your shadow is just your shadow—there's no need to run away from it. There's more time to get on with reality—more time to live and love and to laugh and garden.

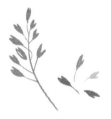

Name and Gain

Too often, we identify with our thoughts and feelings—and by "identify," I mean "invest"—so we let them infest us. Mindfulness teaches us to identify or recognize the thought or feeling and not get fixated on it. We don't have to cling to every notion, random idea, or impression; we can let them go and maintain our focus on being real and present in the world rather than being driven or chasing.

You have heard of name and shame; well, this exercise is name and gain. It is recommended in the early days of meditation. In a meditation, if a thought crops up, you recognize it and don't dwell on it; you just return your focus to meditating. Trying to suppress it or feeling guilty that you're thinking it is undoing of calm and focus—the aim of meditation.

If, during a mindfulness exercise, you realize that you're thinking about lunch, it's okay to acknowledge it. Then simply leave the yum and return back to om—or the task at hand. You identify or recognize what is occurring and continue to the next moment—the thought or feeling may travel with you or it may not. It is all training to move beyond—not to dwell but rather to strengthen focus and control beyond "easily distracted."

In a mindful gardening context, you can do it with bodily sensations too. So if your back aches, you can identify that you are feeling a little discomfort and modify your actions—leave the weeding or digging for another day, and move to a different gardening activity. You call it out and move on from it.

It's the same with emotions—with sadness or fear. Call it out, and move beyond it to the next now. The game is to call it out without judgment and let go. This is the flow of moment-to-moment. This is attainment of mindfulness. Mindfulness is not a single now. We often meet it in a moment, but it is carrying the essence of it moment-to-moment that is the real gain.

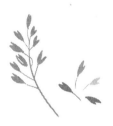

"*Mindfulness isn't just about knowing that you're hearing something, seeing something, or even observing that you're having a particular feeling. It's about doing so in a certain way—with balance and equanimity, and without judgment. Mindfulness is the practice of paying attention in a way that creates space for insight.*"

—Sharon Salzberg

Root Delusion

In Buddhism, there are six root delusions that contribute to an afflicted or nonvirtuous mind: attachment, anger, pride, ignorance, afflicted doubt, and afflicted viewpoint (mindset).

Mindfulness has its origins in Buddhism. Many people today practice a secular sort of mindfulness, but the more we practice, the more we empty ourselves of prejudices, aberrant thinking, and delusion—the more we fill up with being.

In being—in living a less thought-cluttered and trigger-emotion–driven life—we can't help but enter a spiritual realm. So whether it's for relaxation, improved quality of life, better mental health, and so on—no matter the intention, becoming more mindful has a spiritual dimension. We cannot delude ourselves on that score.

Without Dichotomies

When you spend your time in the natural world, you begin to see that everything is interconnected—that everything affects everything else and nothing is separate. We witness how weather and climate impact growth, how soil health impacts crop yield and plant health, and how a harsh winter may dip the bird population and have a subsequent negative effect with some pest populations later in the year.

Sure, it is a cause-and-effect relationship, but it is also a very neat example of nondualism, which is the spiritual concept found in Hindu, Buddhist, and Taoist traditions. It proposes that everything is interconnected, everything affects everything else, and nothing is separate.

In becoming more mindful, we move to being not separate; we interexist with the reality of our self—and our being—in the reality of the now. There is no contradiction or friction; there is an at-oneness. Concepts such as "I," "mine," and "other" are transcended. There is but one unity out of which all of existence arises—or as the Taoists may say, there is only the way.

Mindfulness is the way to reveal this truth or "state of consciousness." As mindful gardeners lost in our work and passion, we become embodiments of "undifferentiatedness"; garden and gardener are in union—the natural world and our natural self are manifest without dichotomies. The ultimate reality presents itself.

Interbeing

Interbeing is a Buddhist concept modernized and explored in the works of author and Buddhist monk Thich Nhat Hanh. It stems from insight into the reality of nature or, indeed, the nature of reality that all things are interconnected. We witness it in the symbiosis of the natural world, in the development of human society, and in cause and effect.

As gardeners, we "inter-be" with our garden. It "inter-bes" with our attention and actions and with the seasons, the pollinators that visit it, the makeup of its soil, and so on. All things exist together. Together is the greater one. The "all" in the "one." There is no duality. We are intertwined. In being, we are more than. In being, we connect with the all.

Mindfulness may help us separate from emotions and suffering—empty the negative. But it connects us to life and reality—to the reality of life and to the life humming within reality. It fills with positivity—it gifts clarity. When we are mindful, we not only bring presence to our being; we bring that to all beings.

Nature Is Interactive and Connective

We step into the garden, and we are home. "Home" is a psychological connection as much as a location. Our neural pathways fire up myriad connections, and we interact with the space and its stimuli and associations. At home, we are safe to be our true selves—to drop the mask and etiquette and be. We may have to become someone else during the workday, but here we are, free from compartmentalizing. Here we merge into and with our surroundings. Here we are interactive and connective just by witnessing the garden.

The bee pollinates a flower. The bird rests on a branch. The spider traps a fly. The pond or lake is filled with water that rains from the evaporation of water from the same or another pond or lake. The sun shines; the grass grows. The breeze stirs; a seed is dispersed. Interaction is everywhere. Connect with that now.

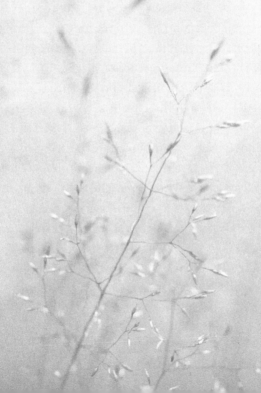

"The highest reward for a man's toil is not what he gets for it but what he becomes by it."

—John Ruskin

Mindfulness Requires Nurture

Just like a garden, mindfulness requires nurture. Just as you feed soil to increase its microbes, by continually adding mindful moments to your life, you feed and strengthen neural pathways that enhance mindful perception and activations of more mindful experiences. You create a positive loop, an upward spiral. Mindfulness modifies the middle prefrontal lobe area of the brain, which regulates intuition, self-insight, and fear modulation.

But just like a newly germinated seed or sapling, mindful practice must be nurtured until it can thrive on its own. Following your breath once a week in a yoga class is not living mindfully. That is not practicing (commitment toward); it is "practicing at" (pretending to be). More is required. You would not plant a few plants, come back later in the year, and expect a garden. No, both a garden and mindfulness require some care to establish.

Care is not a single act; it is repetition. Repetition is a key tenet of living a mindful life; it is not monotonous repetition of tasks and chores but rather glorious returns to elevations of the spirit and clarity of consciousness. In mindful gardening, it is not monotonous repetition of tasks and chores but similarly glorious returns to elevations of the spirit and clarity of consciousness. There is no pretending to be; there is the cultivation of "being."

Mindfulness Is the Nurture

It is regularly deliberated that all transcendental experiences, spiritual awareness, and consciousness awakening are fired in the brain, not in the furnace of the soul. Certainly within the Buddhist tradition from which mindfulness arose, the virtuous path is tread with "clear comprehension"—it is the clarity to see, to know what to do, and to be present in the moment. Enlightenment is truly seeing. Even the Buddha took years to train the brain toward enlightenment. Jesus spoke in parables to engage intellect and heart. Opening the heart may start with opening your mind.

Given that the brain is shaped by external experience as well as contemplative and reactive thought, it is fed from every angle. But where is the nurture? Mindfulness is the nurture. In mindfulness practice, we not only feed but also resonate care into those neural networks—we reshape the pathways of the brain toward responding more to care and positivity, more toward clear comprehension, and more toward flourishing. It may sound like a koan, but mindfulness is the way to mindfulness.

Respond Accordingly

When the soil is warm enough for active growth, active growth happens. When the day length is too short for leaves to photosynthesize efficiently, plants may drop those leaves and conserve energy. Nature signals, and the garden responds accordingly.

In life, we humans often react rather than respond—one is *knee-jerk;* the other is *considered.* Mindfulness helps us attune better to appropriate responses—not to have a rush of blood to the head but rather a flow of awareness from our spirit. This awareness is not wasting energy on anger when loving-kindness will move us more effectively beyond the difficulty—or it's knowing when it is time to put our energies toward growth and experiences and when it is time to let those leaves go.

In practicing mindfulness and living a more positive life, we begin to respond naturally to our own best interests. One may call it cultivating a more refined instinct, but in living more mindfully, our awareness is broadened to what we need in our moment-to-moment existence, and we simply respond accordingly.

This Year's Roses

There are two ways to achieve mindfulness—one is in stillness, and the other in action. So on one hand, you have two paths in, and on the other, there is no excuse for saying you can't get there. If you have picked up this book, then you are already journeying. And that old saying that "life is a journey, not a destination"—well, so, too, with mindfulness.

Mindfulness is a skill you can hone and incorporate into your life. It will enrich the journeying. At first, it is something to experience; then it becomes a way to experience something. Soon it is how you heighten the experience of everything—from making the bed to making a garden to making love to making the bed again.

That may be prepping the rose bed, growing the rose, smelling the rose, pruning the rose, and prepping the bed again for next year's flush of roses. The goal of mindful gardening is learning to enjoy this year's roses fully. May your path be strewn with roses, and may you notice that it is.

"One is wise to cultivate the tree that bears fruit in our soul."

—Henry David Thoreau

Cultivating a Disciplined Mind

Mindfulness is a way of programming the mind to be more disciplined. That makes it a great spiritual tool but also a great psychological tool. Through mindfulness we can master our reactions to emotions and stressful occurrences. We can take control. We can face reality with resilience and with our fully switched-on self.

Mindfulness requires discipline, and mindfulness is a discipline. You don't acquire it; you practice it. In practicing, you enter it. As gardeners, we already know something about discipline; we know that if we don't weed, water, and tend with diligence, we won't have a garden for long. Even without knowing it, the garden has been training you to be a more disciplined being. The garden has been preparing the seed bed for your mindfulness. Go flourish in it.

The Ins and Outs of It

We already looked at how the starting point to mindfulness can be a breath exercise. "Following your breath" means being conscious of your breathing pattern and tuning in to it as a way of tuning out thoughts and other distractions—from surroundings to physical pain. It means being conscious of your breathing as a way to awaken your presence and simply notice thoughts and not attach to them. Following the breath is following a well-established path to more mindful living. It is one that we mindful gardeners will repeatedly sow.

So find a comfortable place in the garden or wherever you are right now, and breathe. Simply inhale and exhale. Feel the rhythm in and out—how your lungs expand and contract, how the air moves through your nostrils and mouth. If a thought arises, let it go and return to focusing on experiencing the breathing rhythm—you can think "inhale" on the in and "exhale" on the out—like a mantra. Or you can feel the in and the out as an experience. For any thoughts that arise, let them go and return your focus to breathing, in and out, in and out. This is breath awareness, this is conscious breathing, this is meditative breathing—this is mindfulness.

By doing this, you are not considering what's next or what happened on that Netflix show last night—

you are in the moment of breathing and being alive to the experience. You are in the now of it. The more one practices this, the less grip those distracting thoughts will have. Soon, starting to breathe consciously will switch on a more focused self—a mind less full of chatter and a more mindful moment-to-moment experience.

Return to your breath often, and you will cultivate a strong presence. It is easy to do while the watering can is filling, as you water, while you mow, or when you plant. It's as easy as breathing. It is breathing only with attentiveness. You are not multitasking by breathing and watering—you are bringing mindful breath and thus a mindful self to the moment of watering. You are simply watering with a mindful presence in play.

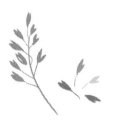

Coming to Your Senses

When we engage a sense, we open up to experiencing. The sense and the sensation make it real. Coming to your senses as a means to mindfulness is as fundamental as using your breath. Throughout this book, we have an opportunity to sow all the varieties of this seed, but for now let's read the details on the packet.

You can shift your mind's focus from thoughts by bringing yourself to your senses.

You can go outside and feel the warmth of the sun on your face. You can let yourself go with the experience; become present to soaking up the pleasantness.

You can smell a flower or taste an edible berry. The trick is to live and enjoy the moment, and the experience will resonate in the brain more than any brain chatter.

Coming to your senses is automatic mindfulness—it is experience, not thought.

Pick a sense—touch, taste, sight, smell, or sound. Now step into the garden, and experience it there.

Sensation Awareness Is Mindfulness

The activation of sensation awareness can successfully trigger your mindful awakening. Coming to your senses is the route to experience, and it offers both grounding and transcendence. Almost like a Zen koan, it takes you out of yourself and into yourself.

Sensation awareness is both an interface with reality and a portal to higher consciousness. Coming to your senses or mindfully engaging with your sensory perception is a true experience. It is how we evolved to read reality, to interoperate it. That split second of smelling, seeing, touching, tasting, or hearing is how we understand and participate with the world around us. Mindful engaging with our sensory perception makes the act of smelling or seeing a moment of being—we are not just receiving information; we are being alive and alert to it.

Sure, we are receiving all this information from the real world anyway, but our minds often run that program on low priority as our pressing thoughts demand more attention. Being mindful turns up the power on receiving the real and, in doing so, turns up our power to experience it—to really be present in that moment. In this moment. Now. Wow.

Following your breath is sensation awareness. Mindfully walking is sensation awareness. Conscious eating is sensation awareness. Gardening is full of sensory activation. Our senses are heightened in the act and actions of gardening as well as by just being in the garden. That, too, is a way to experience its stimulations: those sights, sounds, textures, fragrances, and even tastes.

Why not truly be there? Go engage with it right now. Pick a sense, and seek out the experience.

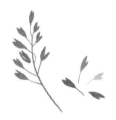

"*Each of us is an artist of our days; the greater our integrity and awareness, the more original and creative our time will become.*"

—John O'Donohue

Bodily Awareness

Mindfulness is not just a mode of the mind; it is of the body and of the spirit too. There are many ways we can use the body to be open to mindfulness—to flower in its presence. In this book, there are prompts for sitting and walking meditations—to yoga, tai chi, and raking like a Zen monk; this is inhabiting our body and bringing it into the now. There is no fantasizing now, conjuring it in the mind like a daydream. There is but presence of mind to reality—when we use our bodies, we are physically grounded in the moment.

Sure, it is nice to think happy thoughts to alleviate stress. But how powerful is it to feel your breath fill your lungs or the air on your skin or the stretch of a limb, right there in the experience of the life of the moment—at the beating heart of it? Bringing your body to mindfulness is as important as bringing your mind to it. It's so important that it is step one of the Satipatthana Sutta—where the Buddha advocates awareness of the body in the body as the first of the four foundations of mindfulness.

Knowing your body and how it reacts to stimuli—to stress and to reward—is a key insight into your own psychological makeup. It may strengthen your practice, and it may give you areas to work on. Knowing your body's reactions—and getting in tune with its physicality and its way of being a bridge of senses to your inner self—is like knowing what aspect your garden is facing and what your soil is like. It is the ultimate foundation against rash errors; it is a solid understanding.

As gardeners, we are physical beings—we flex that body a fair bit, and we flex those senses a fair bit too. So much that bodily awareness can all become background noise. Notice your body today. Hear it again. Bring your attention to sensations that arise as you garden. We are corporeal. Be corporeal. We can be both corporeal and spiritual—there is no separation. When we meditate, it is our whole being that meditates. When we mindfully garden, it is our whole being that gardens.

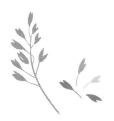

The Body Scan

Apopular mindful exercise is the body scan—a practice where you check in with your body and bring your attention to it in a systematic way. It is a way of slowing down the pace before a meditation. It is a way to check in with the self at the end of a long day. It is a way to take control when distressed. It is a way to get some "awareness of the body in the body"—a prime pillar of mindfulness.

I like the body scan because you can do it on a crowded train, in the garden, or in an elevator as easily as in a mediation room. For the first few times, you might want to do it sitting in a chair, lying on your bed, or in an undisturbed location. As a meditation, it is generally practiced as a ten-to-fifteen-minute exercise. But after a few attempts, you can find a duration that suits you best or modify it to meet your needs. A two-minute body check-in might turn a crowded elevator or escalator jaunt into a positive opportunity for mindfulness, whereas a long commute on a bus, train, or plane may be more suited to a twenty-minute exercise. Mindfulness is being of purpose, but it can suit your purpose.

You can do a body scan standing, sitting, or even lying down. It is a simple noticing exercise. Whatever position you have adopted, start by noticing your posture. Are you standing, sitting, or lying down? Bring your attention to the shape you make, and become aware of the frame of your body. Inhale. Exhale. Notice your body in its physical realm—how the ground is beneath your feet, your solidity in standing, how the chair supports your buttocks and back, or how lying on the bed holds up your body. If you notice a physical sensation or have a thought response like "my neck is stiff," "my feet are tired," or "my shoulders are relaxed," just notice—don't judge. Inhale. Exhale. Your mind is aware of your corporality now; you are bringing awareness to being of a body. Next you will bring your attention through the body.

You can do it from head to toe or toe to head; it doesn't matter which direction. The idea is a systematic scan of the whole body—a gentle sweep and check-in with the parts that make the whole. I often do it standing, so I commence with my feet. You can wiggle your toes to bring your mind there. Become aware of your toes, then bring your attention to your feet and notice any sensation, ache, numbness, or tingling—notice, but do not judge or go into the sensation. Next, move to the ankle and repeat the process. Next to the shin and then the knee; spend a little time noticing and experiencing each section. Next to the thigh, the buttocks, the lower back, and right up to your neck. You can scan your fingers to your shoulders and then to the head. Notice. Experience. Be present to the body and its parts. End by bringing your attention back to the entire body, its posture, its solidity, and its sum of parts. Inhale. Exhale. Take a moment to come back to the room, and then continue your day.

If you choose, you can make this exercise a relaxation scan. You can allow that noticed sensation or any tension present in the body part to cool or soften. This systematic "attention giving" to each section of the body, infusing it with loving-kindness and intended relaxation, is also good practice. The two options are equally valid. Both sharpen your attention capacity; both bring your body into the now.

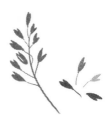

Fired Up

Canadian neuropsychologist Donald Hebb (1904–1985) laid down the maxim "Neurons that fire together wire together." Neuroscientists and psychologists agree that neurons are costrengthened if they co-occur. We evolved to make associations, and it's how prejudices and habitual reactions occur. If fire burns our fingers, we learn a good lesson: that touching fire co-occurred with feeling the burn—"fire + burn" means "fire = burn." And soon we have associations for fire: good for cooking and bad for touching.

Our experience—and the feelings and thoughts that arise with it—connect and embed. This can be the issue with mental health, where we misfire some connections and develop associations with depression, doubt, addiction, attention-seeking, shying away, and all the other obstacles to experiencing the world with peace of mind.

So the more you dwell on pain and suffering, the more you program yourself to be receptive to it—to connect with misery. The more you hear that you are stupid or bad or sinful, the more you deepen the negative input to your perception of self. Sometimes it is not enough to break the toxic relationship; it is vital to clean up the toxic spill. Mindfulness is a pathway to deprogram "self." Mindfulness cleans the spill.

Beyond deprogramming, mindfulness is a way to fire up positive emotions, wellness perception, and spiritual grounding with everyday reality. Mindfulness is truly something to get fired up about.

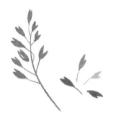

Do More of What You Love

Within the threshold of a neuron firing, our emotions are fixed at a cellular level. Thoughts and words strengthen synaptic connection. We hardwire emotions to experiences. We not only play the story over and over to become the narrative and the narrator, but we feel it as real as well. Just as we can attach to pain and suffering, so, too, can we attach to joy and peace. This is why positive affirmations work so well for many. This is why inspirational quotes pepper this book.

But it is not just about a snappy saying as shorthand for realization of a truth. It is about getting practical with the truth—putting it to use. Bringing it and doing with it. The truth is that the more you enjoy the garden, the more you will perceive and experience enjoyment from the garden—the more being a gardener will bring you to your true being, devoid of pain and suffering, or at least imbued with more joy and peace.

By becoming more of happiness, you become more of love—by being more of love and happiness, you radiate joy and serenity. We should all do more of that. You can garden your soul, but you can also garden for your soul. You can even garden with soul—fire that up. Live it. Love it. Really live it; really love it.

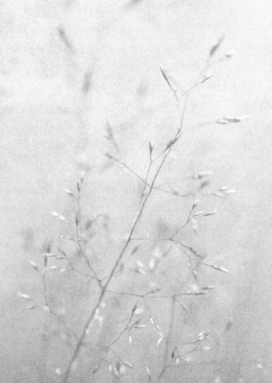

"Zen practice in the midst of activity is superior
to that pursued within tranquility."

—Hakuin Ekaku

The Negative Clearance Trick

As every gardener knows, when you rake a fine tilth over the surface of your soil in order to sow your ornamental or vegetable seed, you can turn up to the surface some weed seeds and they, too, can germinate within your fresh sowing. You can end up with more corn poppy than corn or more nettle than nasturtiums.

You can get discouraged by this, so some gardeners pull a trick to clear the weed seed out first. They rake the ground a week before they intend to sow the crops, allowing the weeds to surface, germinate, and expend their energy into new growth. Then they hoe them off before sowing their profitable seed. We are not called *Homo sapiens* (wise humans) for nothing.

Clearing the negative is not encouraging or indulging in negative thinking; it is seeing the weeds for what they are—unproductive. And no matter how well you tend your garden, there is always the possibility of a newly sprung weed. You may cultivate compassion and rational understanding, but you are not immune to a twinge of anger around social injustice; you don't have to feed it— just see it for what it is whenever it sprouts.

Often when you start a healing or self-dedicating task, your mind's turbulence or socialized psychology can turn up weed thoughts and disincentives: *Is this right for me?*

Can I do this? I am hopeless. Am I wasting my time? How am I going to keep this up? Let all that arise, then hoe each one off. Now you are free to sow—to sow the positive: *It is right for me. I can do this. This is the best use of my time.* Positive affirmations, yes, but also the truth.

We have a natural inclination toward a negative bias, but with mindfulness, we can also sow a positive bias—and, yes, it will thrive like a garden of all the ages.

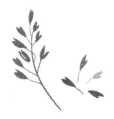

Weeding the Negative Bias

Evolution has provided our minds with a negative bias: a caution reflex—to "think before you leap," in case the gap between this side of the chasm and the green grass on the other side is one stride too far and we fall to our death. Those who ran and jumped without taking the time to think or at least build up some "running momentum" got quickly removed from the gene pool. The worriers hung around and multiplied.

So doubting or having some "hang on a minute" thoughts is a good thing—except when they are not so much life-or-death scenarios but rather intrude on a life in pursuit of being fulfilled or, worse, make a life unfulfilled. We can learn to witness and even appreciate those butterflies in the belly or the "no way" thought but also see beyond—to where the rope bridge across is a better option.

We don't have to weed out every unenthusiastic thought—some of them are more wildflowers than weeds. Don't fret, because mindfulness gifts the clarity to know the difference.

Recognizing a Helpful Weed

Like most gardeners, I weed my garden as diligently as Sisyphus about his business. But I have learned over the years that nettles attract ladybugs, and they eat their fill every day of pest aphids. I know that the dock leaf that can grow beside them will cure me of the sting of a nettle, in case I fancy some nettle soup and have not mindfully or carefully picked. I see the bees on the buttercups. I know that dandelion leaf is as good in a salad as my cultivated lettuce is. So I intentionally refrain from weeding a corner.

I see the usefulness in that weedy patch. It reminds me of discernment, judiciousness, nonjudgment, loving-compassion, gratitude, clear comprehension, interbeing, and much more. I let it be, and it lets me be more.

Paying Attention

Mindfulness is about honing our focused attention—it is all about how we pay attention and to what we give (or don't give) our attention. In mastering our attention, we master our productive selves and create the space for our spiritual selves to flourish. Paying attention is the price of not enduring a life of constant distraction and never truly living any of it.

Increasingly, the modern world orients itself and us toward easy access information and technology—regularly updated 24/7. There is potential for it to be a good thing, but currently, it and we seem to be more at ease with it being all about entertainment and commerce—the two great distractions. Mindfulness existed and was used thousands of years before all this new input. If there was need then, then, wow, is there need now.

All these distractions are a mind full, and mindfulness is not mindless (or mind-deprived). No, it is a mind more fully present—to whatever you choose to be present to. Controlling our own attention is not just the how but the why of mindfulness. It is an essential skill to master to live a life. Attention is more than concentration given to perform a task; it is how we connect with the world around us and with our own being. It is a skill we already have but perhaps do not notice or appreciate much—because we're too often automatically engaged.

This book is about coming into the room with your attention—or, indeed, being in the garden with it. Mindfulness will make your attention bloom.

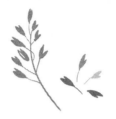

"There is no past, no future; everything flows in an eternal present."

—James Joyce

The Payoff of Attention

Mindfulness is about honing how and to what we pay attention, but there is a great dividend—a taxing break: a break from what taxes our physical energies and higher motivations. With mindfulness, we can have a pleasant experience in an unpleasant environment. The environment may be taxing or draining to our energies, but we can shift our energies—we can shift our terms of focus.

So you may be on a packed train, and instead of dwelling on the claustrophobic atmosphere, you can choose to enter the now of a body scan or do some breath following. Instantly, you are taken out of the sardine can and back into the ocean. You can swim free.

Mindfulness is not only about pleasant experience; it is about a quality of experience, but it can be availed of to change the perception of bad experiences. Mindfulness is about choosing which experience we give our time to— what we do with our now. The more we pay attention and hone our mindfulness muscles—while weeding or smelling a rose—the more it pays off when we need our attention to help us out of a bad spot. It is not running away; it is owning the experience. And if we need to modify it, so be it—wear a nose guard if tending to the compost heap hurts your nostrils. Wear the guard, but finish turning the heap.

The Power of Transformation

Creating a garden is an act of alchemy—it is not just the transmutation of soil and place into a flourishing oasis of vibrant life but also an elevation of spirit and soul in a glorious act of determination and will. You could say that making a garden with all the effort and energy required will make or break you. But it never really breaks; it always makes.

It makes for change; we are transformed by our endeavors. We hone our visual and attentive acuity. We hone our self-expression, and we sharpen our understanding of our true selves. We find our human nature and our divine light in the garden. We are altered by it as we alter it.

We, too, grow and thrive and find our natural groove. We find a home in its ever-changing rhythms, and we are grounded, not perturbed, by its ever-motion. We move with it in full vibrancy; we and it are life in motion. From moment to moment, we are—that is how to be. That is the natural mindfulness every gardener is gifted.

Go Smell a Rose

The story goes that Aphrodite, born on the turbulent sea, turned to face land and, resplendent in her nakedness and assured of her purpose, strode ashore and picked a rose. What does that tell us?

Well, the goddess of love, the queen of sensuality, picked a rose—a plant with a strong perfume. She didn't just pick a pretty flower; she selected a sense to be her first earthly experience. Roses are always inhaled; they give off their fragrance even before you lean your nose in. Aphrodite strode ashore and inhaled perfume—a true sensual act, an immediate grounding in the natural world, and an action of becoming real in the real world. She picked a rose. We have been growing them, picking them, gifting them, and, importantly, smelling them ever since.

Go smell one now, for it will trigger pleasure receptors that are hard to maintain a middle distance from. Immerse yourself in it—let it be a sensual experience. Be fully present to it. Let it awaken your sense of smell. Let it awaken your appreciation of life. Let it awaken a pure moment. Go smell a rose—I dare you.

Go Mow the Lawn

Mowing the lawn can be an active meditation—with singularity of purpose, you can mow like a Zen monk or simply be a more mindful gardener. So bring your full attention to the task at hand—do it, and do it well. Be present to it. Be diligent in it.

A job well done is its own reward, but some jobs have hidden rewards. Mowing the lawn is a treat to the amygdala and the hippocampus—the regions of the brain responsible for emotional recognition and response as well as memory and attentiveness. How? Well, the smell of freshly cut grass stimulates a sense of well-being and relaxation by deactivating the body's stress chemistry and suppressing brain stress receptors.

Mowing the lawn should never be a stressful chore, and even if it begins as such, it ends differently. Mowing the lawn is an opportunity to match brain chemistry to intent and fully embrace the now of well-being and serenity. Love the lawn you care for. It loves you back.

Go Gather Rainwater

Tap water can contain chlorine and other filtration chemicals that are not exactly helpful for plant growth and health. Of course, you can let your watering can or bucket sit overnight so that the chlorine evaporates. Some domestic water supplies can be mineral-rich, often called hard water, which is not ideal for the longevity of healthy plants, especially ericaceous plants. Some mineral salts can be removed by boiling and cooling the water, but this is not a sustainable practice. So a loving-kindness to plants and the planet would be collecting rainwater—which is a soft water suitable for all plants—and using it in the garden.

It may be a dedicated water butt, or it may be a tank or pond filled from a roof spill-off system. It may even be simply putting a few buckets out whenever it rains. This sort of doing is expression of and acting on your caring nature; it is the cultivation of diligent concern. A saying attributed to the Buddha that I often ponder while in the garden is "Think not lightly of good, saying, 'It will not come to me.' Drop by drop is the water pot filled. Likewise, the wise man, gathering it little by little, fills himself with good."

So go gather some rainwater, and in light of interbeing and even karmic interconnectivity, we will fill more than a bucket.

*"When you take a flower in your hand and really look at it,
it's your world for a moment."*

—Georgia O'Keeffe

Good Vibes

In healing circles, it is often espoused that the difference between one form of spiritual or physical matter or manifestation and another is simply a consequence of its vibrational state, and vibrations can be tuned. This is seen in everything from chakra cleansing to flower essences.

We can harvest the garden for health, we can grow our favorite herbal tea, we can make our own flower essences, and we can reap the stimulation of color and fragrance. Much about the garden can alter our mood—much that can have a physiologic reaction. Becoming more mindful, we can look to not just how we grow but what we grow—and all of its marvelous potential.

We can extend good vibes, but we can cultivate them and harvest them too. Gather a bunch of flowers for the kitchen table. Gather a bunch of herbs for tonight's dinner. Bring the good vibes of the garden into other aspects of your life.

Cultivating Calm

Why is it that when someone is asked to conjure an image of a holy person or enlightened being, the image is almost always of a serene being—of someone being serene, be that a cross-legged Buddha attaining nirvana or a kneeling monk in quiet repose? Clearly, the human mind associates tranquility with higher attainment. Perhaps the transcendence of pain and suffering could only be a calmed soul—the ultimate spiritual gift is peace.

Well, that's one projection we got right. Even if it is just shorthand for a greater understanding—even if it took that serenity many years to blossom before the snapshot. Yes, the ultimate gift is peace—the absence of disruption. Mindfulness is about attaining peace—peace of mind, peace of heart, peace of soul. It is the emptying of disruption and negative reactions that is so fulfilling— no wonder the Buddha smiles; no wonder the monk has no air of disharmony.

Mindfulness is about weeding out the disruption and cultivating the calm. Mindfulness embodies decentering, nonattachment, emotion regulation, and clear comprehension: the pillars that support peace—the foundations of your own personal piece of calm. Gardening, with its richness of moments of natural tranquility and its fostering of attention regulation away from personal worries and worldly woes, is a cultivation of our calmer and more controlled and grounded selves.

So smile. Have no air of disharmony. Be of the gift of peace; it is with the gift of your garden.

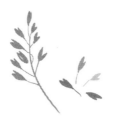

Observing the Nature of Things

Sure, mindfulness can be a relaxation technique—a way to attune to your inner peace. But it is also a means of immediate clarity—not just the development of focus and attainment of acuity but of paying attention to the nature of things and comprehending too.

Mindfulness meditation is observation—the goal is to see our true self clearly; we see it by dropping our beliefs and prejudices. We empty the mind of clutter to uncover what some Buddhist practitioners might call the original mind—a mind freed from attachment. We pay attention with our breath, with our body, with our full and true potential—with our presence.

We observe. We witness. We attend. We recognize. We are the awareness. We are the awe. We are not bound, and we are not separate. That is the wisdom sought, that is the wisdom found, that is the original mind, and that is the original soul. Discover that in the garden today. Let yourself notice the reality of life all around you. Let wisdom, joy, and original self unfold like a leaf or the pop of a flower.

I am reminded of a *waka* (traditional Japanese poem) attributed to Dōgen: "Seeing with ears and hearing with eyes, there is no doubt that the jewel-like raindrops dripping from the eaves are myself."

Cultivating Nonjudgment

As we mindfully garden and engage in the natural world, we foster our natural selves—the nonfilled self, the open self, the true self: our innate spirit. What is the false self? That's the egocentric self: the manifestation of thoughts, emotions, and prejudices or preconceptions—the "I" and "mine" attitude that forces you out of serenity to defend the "I" and "mine" position. Duality.

To cast judgment is to take a side—it is to enter the fray; it is to see the other and to be its opposite. Unity is broken. Harmony is demolished. To judge, you must awaken the self that overly identifies and engages in attachment or the self that separates from the situation with discrimination and verdict. Duality.

Nonjudgment takes you to a place where you can surpass reactive thinking, engage your knowing self, and transcend ego. You can see and acknowledge but remain as the witness, not as judge and jury. It is not a passivity but rather an adoption of a neutral serenity. At-oneness.

When we refrain from judgment, we refrain from the turbulence of the reactive "I" and the disturbance of taking a side; we make peace with the moment and move on from it. Nonjudgment is not just not judging others; it is not judging situations, occurrences within the garden, and ourselves. It is often the hardest ask, but what blooms is beautiful. At-oneness.

Sampajanna

Mindfulness is about the cultivation of a clearer mind—one not overgrown with distraction, pain, and suffering. The more we practice, the more we train the brain for this state of consciousness—for this way of experiencing the reality of the moment. Eventually, instead of trying to become, we have become. We achieve *sampajanna*, or clear comprehension. Awareness arrives. The bud unfurls to flower.

Sampajanna is more than perception; it is not just that you see something for what it is but also that you see and comprehend what needs to be done—or not done—and how that relates to your lived life and the wider world. It is how to be in the moment. It is the unfolding of the awareness of and toward the reality of the moment. It is the repeat flowering of mindfulness.

The lightning bolt of enlightenment, like every other lightning bolt, waits for the perfect climatic and atmospheric conditions to facilitate its occurrence. The Olympic medal is won on the day and all the days leading up to that last second of victory. Patience is rewarded. Effort is rewarded. So in the meantime, we apply patience and diligence.

"*What we plant in the soil of contemplation,
we shall reap in the harvest of action.*"

—Meister Eckhart

The Four Foundations of Mindfulness

Within Buddhism, the four foundations of mindfulness are contained within the Satipatthana Sutta, a training manual for systematically learning how to develop mindfulness.

The first foundation is *kāyā* (body): to pay attention and investigate sensations of the body or how we experience the body.

The second foundation is *vedanā* (sensations/feelings): to notice the tone or "feelings" of experiences—pleasant, unpleasant, or neutral—and not be judgmental or reactive.

The third foundation is *cittā* (mind/consciousness): to bring awareness to the mind's workings—to notice nonjudgmentally any emotions arising within experiences and not jump into mental states as a result.

The fourth foundation is *dharma* (reality): the way of things or of the true reality of the world around you—of bringing your attention and awareness to that.

What if I Just Want to Relax?

Not everyone sees mindfulness as a spiritual undertaking. Some want a handy relaxation technique. Some want mindfulness to improve physical or mental health, and some want to develop a better quality of life, engage with a pastime that helps combat modern stresses, or have a "go-to" in times of distress. That's okay; mindfulness can be a technique as well as a life path. If you just want to use it to relax, then relax. It's all good.

The techniques of mindfulness, although originally spiritual, have secular applications. Mindful gardening can be prayer, or it can be a fuller enjoyment of the garden and gardening activities—either way, it enriches.

Of course, you may only want a garden to sit out in, and then you'll never sit down ever again. It is not that mindfulness and gardening are addictive; it's that they open the portal to being your real self, and that reaches beyond the want of relaxation into the gift of transcendence. Who doesn't want more of that?

Acute Stress versus Chronic Stress

Some people take up mindfulness as a stress reduction technique, and yes, it will bring peace of mind, serenity, and equanimity along with "awake presence." The stronger focus acuity developed by mindful practices can bring your presence to stressful as well as reassuring and relaxing situations—and that's okay. The aim with stress is not to run away from it but rather to harness it or disarm it.

There are two types of stress: the motivational and the destructive—or the acute and the chronic. Acute or motivational stress arises as a direct chemical response to the need to perform—it is the fight-or-flight reaction. The stress brings a concentration or wakefulness, and there are some accelerants in the endorphins and molecules released into the system. This acute stress is a short-term burst of "go get 'em." We evolved with it in order to get things done in a moment of survival, and we kept it to allow motivation and movement in other times of need.

Chronic stress is a different matter; too much of that chemistry is harmful. Chronic or prolonged stress is associated with the development of high blood pressure, brain fog, disruptive thinking, and a weakening of the immune system. Chronic stress is destructive to the body and soul. It is also destructive to brain structure, specifically connections between communicating cells in the hippocampus—the region that regulates emotions, long-term memory, and spatial navigation and has a role in behavioral inhibition, thus keeping us calm and considered rather than reactive and hyperactive.

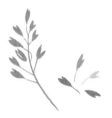

Mindfulness and the Hippocampus

The hippocampus is the part of the limbic region of the brain that governs memory, learning, and emotional responses. The known effects of hippocampal damage manifest in hyperactivity and a diminished capacity to engage behavioral limitations. Hippocampal damage or distortion is regularly noted in stress-related disorders, such as depression and PTSD.

Strengthening neural connections is beneficial for regaining or exerting control over hippocampal functions. In recent years, the "control attainability" of mindfulness has had therapeutic value in this area. What's interesting is that it is not just training to shape—or relearning how to cope with and modify—responses. Rather, the regular practice of mindfulness increases cortical thickness in the hippocampus; it grows control.

"The glory of gardening: hands in the dirt, head in the sun, heart with nature."

—Alfred Austin

Abundant, Exalted, Immeasurable

While synonymous with calmness and composure, equanimity is much more than keeping your cool in a difficult situation. It is more than not throwing your trowel at the neighbor's cat for making a fresh litter tray of your just-sown seeds. It is more than not feeling sorry for yourself when black spot decimates a rose bush. It is beyond staying calm; it is being unaffected. Equanimity could be said to be the goal of mindfulness. Serenity will come soon; equanimity may take more time.

Equanimity is not a stance of cold detachment; it is the embodiment and radiance of being free from attachment and from being drawn into ego and emotional states. It is the way to be unaffected by consequence and bullshit—otherwise known as the eight worldly winds: praise, blame, success, failure, fame, disrepute, pleasure, and pain. It is the even keel in the rough seas of those turbulent things. Praise can go to your head. Blame can hurt your heart. Success can turn your head. Failure can sap your spirit. Fame and disrepute are but fixations. Pleasure is best understood as "pleasure-seeking," which can be not just a distraction from the path but a fool's errand too. As for pain or suffering, that just tethers the self to "I" and "mine" and dualism. Equanimity is the capacity to rise above those winds.

Equanimity is not indifference; it is a loving-compassion toward one's true self—not to react, not to cling, not to get distracted, and not to suffer. It is the choice and freedom not to. The Buddha defined it as "abundant, exalted, immeasurable, without hostility, and without ill-will."

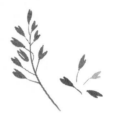

Cultivating Equanimity

In the Buddhist tradition, there are two aspects of achieving equanimity. *Upekkha*, which translates to "to look over," means achieving a viewpoint or perspective to see but not being drawn in. *Tatramajjhattata*, which translates to "the middle stance of it all," means taking up the position of distance (detachment) from the event unfolding. It is the inner calm that allows one to not step forward into the fray or turn to run away. It is not a higher moral ground, for there is no judgment; it is simply remaining centered—in the middle, not in the mix.

Nor is it indifference. In the garden, we may take the stance to stake the leaning bush before the winds come, but if they uproot the plant, then equanimity is taking it stoically—and not apportioning blame to the season or to the stake or to your own perceived "failure" to halt or alter the worst outcome. Stuff happens; we don't have to catastrophize it.

It is said that several mental attributes support the development of equanimity. The first is virtue or blame-lessness, which we can take as personal integrity rather than any set of rules about what sort of moral position should be engaged in. In being true to yourself, you bring veracity to the moment. That is, be authentic, not false or blameworthy or blaming. That is, be solid and unmovable in your own quality of being.

After authenticity comes *saddha*, which means being resolute in your spiritual practice. It is also achieved by applying conviction or confidence in your "being." All the mindful gardening and mindful practices thus far have strengthened your resolve, and you can be assured of that. It is not pride; it is confidence. It is faith.

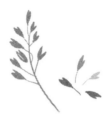

To Look at a Flower

Gardening can be an all-consuming pastime, but within the garden, we can be devoured by love and awe too.

To look at the simple beauty or intricate majesty of a flower is to lose oneself to the moment of it—to be at one and nothing in a single move. There is no need to pluck or search for a vase; look at the plant, how it sings from its natural place, how at home it is in its environment—radiant and resonant. Yeah, looking at a flower is a surefire way of forgetting the travails of the world or the troubles of yourself.

Rare is the answer *just look*—but rather *wait, just look*.

Nature Has Its Own Nature

Too many gardeners are engaged in a battle, if not all-out war, with the natural order of things in order to bring order to their garden. But does the lawn really need to be a billiard table? Do the flower beds have to be so regimented? We can be freer in our approach; we can choose to garden with nature, not attempt to dominate it. We can be more accepting of nature as indomitable. Why waste energy fretting the odd weed or overblown flower?

Nature has its own nature, and it is wonderful to behold. We can of course continue to weed, cultivate, and apply horticultural skill, aiming to create and interact. But we can embrace the spirit of nature in our garden and be less precise and stressed about a pictured perfection—and instead rejoice in all the aspects. Overblown flowers are as real and beautiful as burgeoning buds.

Mindfulness brings with it patience, acceptance, and loving-kindness—it makes that seed bed receptive, but what blooms is also joy. So rejoice in all the aspects—that's only natural too.

Going to Seed

A plant going to seed is fulfilling its destiny—it is going forth and multiplying. It is in its moment of its lifecycle. It is in its now. It is being as it is to be.

As mindful gardeners, we make movements toward being what it is to be. We will always have the urge to garden, but it's okay on some days or in certain situations to do nothing and let it be. We can meet the garden in its now.

A large part of Taoism is nonstriving. Acceptance is nonstriving. The tao of mindfulness is to become effortless. The garden in its flow can remind us to be in our flow. We are not bolting to seed, for we are not stressed—we are simply where we are and in it. Bud, bloom, seedhead—it is all an eternal present; it is all the presence of true nature. Be as you are at whatever stage in life.

"I go to Nature to be soothed and healed,
and to have my senses put together."

—John Burroughs

Greeting the Garden

As you enter the garden, greet it. Extend your respect and appreciation. You can say out loud, "Hello, friend." You can think it quietly in your mind, or you can feel it in your heart. Maybe you want to nod or smile or take a simple inhale of *yes, here we are*. However you want to do it, this is acknowledging the garden as more than a space; it is seeing the habitat—the living thing.

Gardening is participation with the natural world—it is being your living self in a living environment. Greeting the garden is a way to enter into mindfulness as much as it's an appreciative way to enter into the garden. It is a way to state your intentions to connect. It is an expression of gratitude and loving-kindness. It opens the portal. Remember that when you next step through.

Feel It

To garden is to be tactile; tactility is at the heart of it. Sure, we grip the spade. Sure, we cup the apple before we pluck it or the rose before we smell it. Sure, our fingers are often in the earth and sometimes our toes are on the grass, but it is not just a consequence of actions required or a sneaky moment out. Touch, contact, embodied cognition, tactility—that is our interface with the world.

Even before we are born, we receive and respond to tactile signals—we are perceptible to the sensation of the vibration of our mother's heartbeat as it resonates through and is amplified by the amniotic fluid we inhabit; our universe vibrates. It is the first language. It is the first message.

Today as you touch soil, or run your hand over a plant, really feel it. Accept its texture onto your skin; let those sensors resonate, and vibrate it to your heart, to your soul. Hear that message. Be in communication with this universe.

Mow the grass, and feel it. Do tai chi on the lawn, and feel it. Inhale the sky, and feel it. Get outside, and feel it.

Go Taste the Garden

Taste is a sense; it sparks an immediacy of experience. No matter what the flavor—sour or sweet—your taste buds receive it. To realize a taste is to truly experience it. Eating should be more than swallowing fuel or relieving boredom or because it is time. Yes, eating relieves hunger and nourishes the body, but it can be a powerful experience if we allow it to be. Too often, we eat on the go, eat in front of the TV, eat with the ambiance in the way, or eat as an occasion but with too much circumstance—when do we truly taste? To be more mindful, we should taste.

Often, mindful eating is used to familiarize ourselves with healthy eating—to taste is to modify pace, to embrace the meal is to feel fulfilled and satisfied at one sitting. But weight loss or food phobias aside, to mindfully taste is to engage an intrinsic sense and be of our core being. To really taste is to realize and be realized in the moment-to-moment occurrence of it.

You may have a kitchen garden; if not, it is easy to incorporate some herbs in ornamental planters or borders. No matter what style of garden you keep, there is something edible in the garden right now—a mint leaf, a sweet or tart berry, or even a blade of grass. As long as you're sure that it is clean, chemical-free, and nontoxic and that you are not allergic, taste it. You don't have to swallow a plateful; you don't even have to swallow at all. A simple split-second suck or chew, and it will release its flavor.

Bring your attention to that; allow your mouth and your being to notice and register that taste. Foul, fair, or delicious—no matter. It is awakening a sense, it is bringing your focus to the moment now unfolding, you are truly tasting, and you are alive in this moment—and if you followed my rules, you will still be alive in the next.

We see the garden, we hear it, we smell it, and we touch it daily. How often do we taste it? It is well worth having a garden that can activate all five senses and, in that, unify how we read the world with the story it has to tell. Our senses make sense of the world for us. Get real in your garden—go taste it.

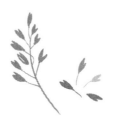

Go Get Grounded

To stop for a moment and stand still is a great way to slow the pace, catch your breath—even follow your breath—and find some inner peace. A standing meditation is as powerful as a sitting meditation.

Gardeners know silence, and we often know true peace, but we may be less used to stillness—there is always something to be done, but in doing for yourself, stillness is rejuvenating. Stillness is recharging the spiritual and mindful batteries. It is pure being. Be it from time to time.

Standing still, feel your feet on the floor surface. Notice the solidity of your legs as they push the weight of your body onto your feet—as the earth takes that weight and supports up. You are firm and present; feel your presence—it is strong, solid, and actual. There is life here. There is connectedness to the solidity of the ground beneath you. You can be a mighty oak in this moment. You can be a resilient gardener in this moment. You can be a human taking a moment. In the moment-to-moment of it, feel your standing strength. Stillness is energy. Stillness is energizing. Stillness is.

"See with your eyes, hear with your ears, taste with your tongue. Nothing in the universe is hidden."

—Tenkei Denson

A Barefoot Connection

There are other potent advantages to standing still, especially if you slip off those shoes and socks. A barefoot connection to the earth is even more rejuvenating. Feeling the texture of the grass, soil, or concrete is coming to your senses, combined with the energy of stillness. Being barefoot is being free, unburdened, and natural. That is psychologically rewarding—that is also spiritually uplifting.

Standing still while barefoot is a way to divest ourselves of not just psychological tensions but also static electricity and physical tension. Walking around all day in shoes and socks creates electrical friction and builds up static electricity in our bodies, which can interfere with bodily functions and our sense of energy, capability, and alertness.

Standing barefoot on your lawn for three to five minutes—take longer if you can—is an ionic detox for your body. It improves the function of your organs and immune system, as well as increasing neuron and synaptic firing. When you connect barefoot to the earth, you allow the earth to change your electrical charge—to ground you again. With the static dissipated, you absorb ample quantities of powerful antioxidant and anti-inflammatory free electrons through the soles of your feet. Not just energizing—health-conferring.

Getting barefoot from time to time is a good grounding in building health and an extra sensory experience to entering the now. It doesn't have to be all standing still. Barefoot tai chi or yoga on the lawn works as a treat too.

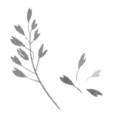

Positive Regard

We gardeners reap such rewards from our gardens. Before we even get an edible harvest or can cut flowers for the table, an herbal tea, or a curative plant, we get healthy fresh air. We get vitamin D from the sun. We get the boost of achieving and the pleasure or distraction of doing something we enjoy. A day of hard labor or a day of gentle puttering about—no matter; the garden cultivates our spirit.

We can think of that from time to time. It is okay to think in a mindful life—a mindful life brings clarity of thought. It also brings good emotions to the surface. Mindfulness is not eradication of emotions—we can have positive regard. Today, extend positive regard to your garden. Extend positive regard in how you tend the garden. Water lovingly. Weed lovingly. Pick, plant, prune, or potter lovingly.

If "lovingly" is too strong for you just yet—then how about "with simple appreciation"? That's the seed of love.

To Look at a Leaf Anew

The garden is full of foliage, and the foliage can be as dramatic and appealing as any flower—so much so that many gardeners grow for foliage and deeply appreciate all the aesthetics of shape, color, and texture. But to look at a single leaf is an exercise in conscious observation. You can leave it on the plant but take it into your hand, or you can pluck it and hold it up to the light. It is not any particular vantage point that is important; it is truly looking—to really see.

At first one may look at the leaf and see its shape, color, and texture—but really looking is to bring your full attention to all its facets. Bring your attention to its shape; fully see that. Now notice any texture that may be present; draw your attention to any fine detail. Drink in its color, its vibrancy. Look at it as if for the first time. Explore its dimensions. Bring your presence to its presence. Be present to it; it is present to you.

It is amazing how conscious observation can ignite renewed appreciation for items that have become background or mundane. By mindfully looking, we fire up not only the pattern recognition section of the brain but wire it with deep appreciation and even awe. Be in that moment.

A Garden for Now

All gardeners want to build or create a garden to be in and be proud of. It is not just a creative action; it is a place of continual creative actions. Sure, we want a garden with paving, boundaries, vistas, interest points, and so on—all the trappings of permanence—but we know, too, that it is shifting, evolving, and transitory. There is impermanence in our Eden. Such is life or, should I say, "That's life"—because that is life.

The garden is how it is now. It is always how it is now; it is forever in the reality of its place within the season and in the context of your attentive self—how much or how little you have tended it lately. It was a different beast two months ago; it will be different again in three months' time. The garden does not stand still, even when you do. It simply is what it is in each moment. Pausing to appreciate the moment is mindfulness. Moving on to mindfully tend the needs of the garden in the manner it is in now is seeing the reality—is participation with reality.

This is the mindful gardener's life—how rich.

"*If you want others to be happy, practice compassion.
If you want to be happy, practice compassion.*"

—His Holiness the Dalai Lama

Loving–Kindness

As gardeners, we regularly extend loving-kindness—it is the nurture reflex we have cultivated ever since we sowed that first seed, brought home that first plant, or learned at a parent's or grandparent's knee how to water a new plant or plant a spring bulb. Expressing loving-kindness outward is easy.

Expressing loving-kindness inward may not be so easy. We gardeners tend be hard taskmasters on ourselves, and while we may forgive the slug or pigeon, we may not forgive forgetting to net or lay a beer trap. We are human. "Only human" is the phase often used. We can strive to be more, but why not love your humanity as it is right now? You can love your perfected self tomorrow, but right now, you are already doing well. If you were not aware of your flaws, you wouldn't be human. You would have no awareness skills.

So while you may have sent off for an upgrade, accept yourself now. You are not doing too badly—send a little loving-kindness within.

Vipassana

The aim of mindfulness is clarity. Throughout this book, the prompt "to notice" arises. To notice is to come to the reality of the moment. That, too, is the aim of mindfulness; that is clarity of experience, that is clarity of comprehension, and that is clarity of life in real time—in being present.

Vipassana is a Pali word for insight, clarity, or clear awareness. *Vipassana* is a form of meditation that derives from Theravada Buddhism. It is not a concentration meditation, where one focuses on the breath or a mantra to regulate thought patterns and train the brain and mind to focus better. It is an insight meditation, where one simply observes and trains the mind, body, and spirit to truly see. *Vipassana* can be translated as seeing the world as is. This is the clarity of experience—to see the reality of it.

A simple *Vipassana* meditation can be to observe your breathing pattern—is it long, deep, short, or shallow? No judgment, no modification. Just observe what it is—the reality of how you are breathing right now. This is bringing your attention to the reality of this moment, of this life action—this is observing truth. There is only the observance of—and no reaction to—the true nature of your breath in this moment. There is no emotional response—

just witnessing. No attachment—just being there with it in its reality. Pure presence.

The flowering of this type of meditation is a strengthening of not just observational capacity but of participation in reality as it is. Looking consciously at a flower and seeing it without judgment is flexing this clarity. Smelling the fragrance of a rose or a culinary herb is accepting the reality of its scent. Awareness of your skin in the outside atmosphere is being present to the ambient temperature of now. All of this is not just seeing and knowing the world as it is; this is being in the world as it is. Pure presence.

Mindfulness is great to empty your mind of pain and suffering, but it is great, too, to fill your being with true reality. Pure presence.

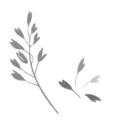

To Consciously Water

You can water like a *Vipassana* exercise and bring your attention to the process of witnessing the watering—no judgment or reaction, just being present to the watering activity. This is to consciously water. This is to mindfully water. Observing the reality of the activity, being in the reality of the moment.

Be it an indoor potted plant, a hanging basket, or a section of the garden, go water something now. Water with presence.

To Consciously Tend a Border

To tend a border requires not just creative expression or an eye for what looks good together but also horticultural understanding of the plants you grow. To put a plant in the wrong place or wrong soil type can be its early demise—so life-or-death is on the line. To tend a border requires aptitude.

To tend a border requires understanding the needs of the plants in your care—how often to water, how deep or shallow its roots might go, how hungry a feeder it may or may not be. It requires commitment to care. Not engaging just your nurturing self but also your attentive self. You must be present and aware when tending a border, or you may miss the first signs of rust, mildew, or other potential calamities. You must be vigilant to pests and to techniques that deliver the best outcomes for your plants—deadheading, pruning, division, feeding, and watering. A garden is a commitment and one of a lifetime—in duration and possibly even magnitude. There is a union of interaction and interdependence. You both thrive for the experience. It will require patience, a little sacrifice, a lot of hard work, and moments of pure joy.

To tend a border is an intimate engagement with life—to do it mindfully is to live to the fullest.

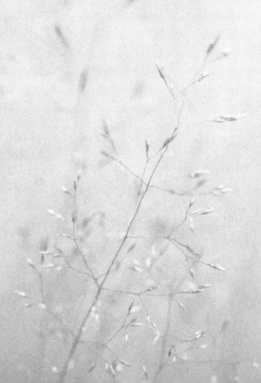

"*Rather than being your thoughts and emotions,*
be the awareness behind them."

—Eckhart Tolle

To Rake Like a Zen Monk

In Zen garden design, those sand or gravel expanses represent water or, more specifically, the sea, which is ever-changing yet consistent, just like life. There's a metaphor—a lesson to the monks who tend the space and civilian onlookers to gain insight from viewing and comprehending. These gardens are minimalistic—often just rock gravel and moss, occasionally a miniature shrub in a tree shape—but they were designed for more than spiritual symbolism and microrepresentations of the macro. They were designed for monks to tend—for monks to daily reshape that ever-changing but consistent ocean.

The practice of raking is an active meditation—there is both doing and being. It embodies some key Zen attributes: "Do one thing," "be diligent," and "be of it." As a task, it is one ask; create a pattern—focused attention is required. In Zen monasteries, a monk's work was a way to realize *satori* (comprehension of reality), which calls for mindful participation.

The monastic raking is a specific technique that takes skill to master; it is commenced on a breath and follows a honed movement to breath syncopation or patterning. Beyond diligence, this firmly grounds the body and the mind in union for the task at hand. This demands your presence; you can't be not of it. You have to be there with your full self.

The Zen gravel ocean is a mandala. It embraces and celebrates impermanence. It embraces and celebrates change. Reshaping today and getting up tomorrow to do it all over again brings Buddhist philosophy about impermanence and transition into play. Surrendering to the ever-changing but consistent nature of reality is acceptance of reality. It is realization of truth; it is liberating.

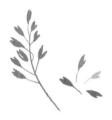

To Really Rake the Lawn

In a mindful meditation, even if that is a dynamic one such as raking the lawn as a mindful engagement, it is not just about relaxed states of mind and a sense of well-being and accomplishment—although that follows. It is about being present and communicating that presence to the universe. There is no ego in this; you are not shouting over the fence, "Look how well I am doing." No, now in your mindful state, you are both channeling positive vibes and sending them into the world.

You rake the lawn to clear it of falling leaves, to gather up the clippings of the last mow, to scarify it of moss, or to otherwise refresh and energize it. We are interconnected as life. As you refresh and energize your lawn, so you energize and refresh your own self and soul.

I am reminded of the eighteenth-century Japanese Zen master Hakuin Ekaku, who espoused, "Zen practice in the midst of activity is superior to that pursued within tranquility." You know, in this instance, the sweat on the brow is a good thing; the hard work is its own reward.

Go rake the lawn, and scarify it if you need an excuse—but be present to it. Do that one thing that is everything.

Become Still as a Tree

When going full steam ahead in the garden, it is not good just for the knees and back to take a break; it is also good for the soul to find a little stillness from time to time. If you need a cause to pause, then nothing beats a stillness meditation.

Attune to your mindful breathing. Then, with your eyes open or closed, bring your attention to the solidity of your physical self. You can do this as a visualization and imagine yourself as a tree—rooted and yet free to extend your canopy toward the sky, fully alive in the moment. Sturdy, still, majestic.

Now simply embody stillness, embody strength, and embody at-oneness. There you have it. That's the fundamental truth. Exhale it out.

Listen to the Bees

We evolved our senses to strengthen our experience of the world. The garden is rich in sensual cues and pleasures—not least how we hear it: the rustle of trees, the swish of ornamental grasses, and the trickle or cascade of a water feature.

Bees are the sound of summer, and their hum may be as welcome as birdsong to some. It is not just the sound of good weather or the soundtrack to blossoming flowers but also the noise of the engine of nature. Bees pollinate our plants and trigger fruiting and seed production. The hum we hear is that of industry.

Bring your attention to the sounds of those bees busy about your garden, busy with its upkeep. They, too, are the gardeners that tend this space. Listen with attentiveness. Listen with appreciation.

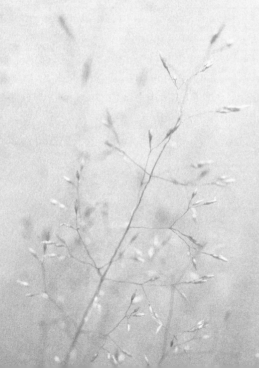

"*Getting in touch with true mind is like digging deep in the soil and reaching a hidden source that fills our well with fresh water.*"

—Thich Nhat Hanh

Feel the Breeze

The natural world facilitates mindful awareness. Just step out into it. Feel the air on your skin, feel the air as it enters and leaves your lungs, and notice the movement of the foliage. Is there a breeze—how strong is it? Feel for it; don't just look or listen for it. Close your eyes, and let your body sense it. This is focused attention. This is a mindful moment.

You may feel the breeze on your skin; deepen your awareness of how that physically feels. Notice the sensation of a breeze on your skin—it may be a gentle caress or a bit more robust; it may be warming, or it may be chilling. Your skin is reading the environment you live in; your skin is reading the climatic reality of the moment. You are interfacing with the natural world; your skin and the air are meeting.

This is how we evolved to experience the world. You may feel the air move your clothing or hair; pay attention to that experience. This has all happened a million times before, but it is happening right now—indulge in it. Come alive to it—what a truly beautiful experience.

Perspective

As gardeners, we learn that not every seed germinates and most plants won't avoid the attention of slugs—but we keep at it anyway. We become resilient and take the setbacks in stride. It is part and parcel of it. The thing is—do we take the burnt toast or the failed direct debit so well? Well, we can learn to.

For most gardeners, the garden is their life. We do apply the life lessons we learn in it—but the more mindful the moments and the more mindful the intent, then the more we rewire our emotional circuitry and the more we become less personally affected by mishaps in the nongardening parts of our life. Mindful gardening is mindful living. Mindful gardening is knowing that shit happens but being ready to feed the roses.

Day-to-day gardening cultivates the middle way—that equanimity so prized by monks of every perspective. We just learn to get on with it. That becomes our vantage point. We can bring this awareness to all the aspects of our lives. Shaped by our experiences, we have blossomed a good perspective.

The Garden Teaches Managed Attention

There is a lot going on within a garden. It may even contain more than one ecosystem—a pond, a wild meadow patch, trees, ornamental borders, and a kitchen garden. There is upkeep for all of them and the infrastructure too—paving to be kept moss- or weed-free, benches and seats to be kept rot- or rust-free, and trellis or supports to be maintained. Attention and diligence are required. We gardeners learn to pay attention to all areas and prioritize our focus and activities too.

When we step into it, there may be more than one need competing for our attention. We can triage plants into water now, catch before we finish, deadhead now, prune later, remove pests now, and add frost protection before we wrap up. The wind-rocked, newly planted shrub gets priority over a slightly shaggy lawn. The weed about to flower—or, worse, disperse its seed—gets the "next" before the squeaky shed door gets the oiling.

On one level it is common sense, but it's also a catchment of your experience—you know that if you don't water the wilted plant, it could be set back detrimentally or even die overnight. You know that not bringing the tenders in before the heavy frost may mean losses. All this previous experience creates effectiveness. All this repeat effectiveness strengthens our effectiveness response and brings that potential to other aspects of our lives.

People who struggle with efficiency have an issue with prioritizing what needs to be addressed or seeing the forest for the trees. The garden—and its constant elicitation of managed attention—trains a clarity with regard to need and even crisis. We gardeners are fixers. We are prioritizers by nurture and, soon enough, by nature. In a crisis, we quickly spot that, yes, it's a good idea to fire a flare gun, but instead of everybody waving to the horizon and shouting "Help!," it's better if the majority of hands tend to the leaky boat. The longer one stays afloat, the less likely one is to go under before rescue.

In a garden, a workplace, a domestic crisis, or a life-threatening circumstance, with so many stimuli competing for attention, the survival protocol is effectiveness. Part of that is knowing what to do, but a lot of it is seeing clearly. Mindfulness is seeing clearly without panic—mindfulness is focusing your managed attention to the now. When problems arise, managed attention leads to managed action—and that may lead to more than survival of a wilted herb container.

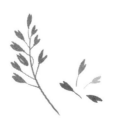

The Practice of Patience

Patience is not always an easy ask, but it is well worth the task and effort of acquiring. The garden teaches patience; seeds take time to germinate, cuttings take time to root, borders and planting schemes take time to establish, and a tree could take your lifetime to mature. Patience is as essential as a trowel. I often think fondly of the Chinese proverb "Patience is a tree with bitter roots that bears sweet fruits." We soon overcome bitterness, as we know what will flourish.

It is often through our patience that we acquire our resilience. It is often through patience that we find our gratitude. It is certainly through patience that we master our mind's workings and bring awareness to fruition. Just like every other mindful skill, the more we practice patience, the more patient we become.

The more we follow our breath, walk with resolve, plant with purpose, water with presence, and generally garden and live with intent, the more we resolve impatience. The more we go with the flow, the more we find our flow—the more we grow a tolerant and enduring spirit.

While patiently waiting on the watering can to fill, we are not really waiting; we are *being while*. While patiently waiting on seeds to germinate, we are *being while*. While patiently practicing, we are fully *being*. Ripening sweet fruits.

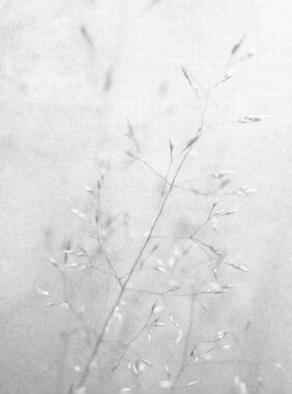

"Ever tried. Ever failed. No matter. Try again. Fail again. Fail better."

—Samuel Beckett

Adapting

If there is one lesson in evolution, it is "adapt and survive." Evolution shows that the overly rigid and the reticent are removable. The natural world has its rhythms and seasons; the secret to surviving and thriving is adapting to each new one—to move with it. In mindfulness circles, we talk a lot about moment-to-moment—because our nows are continuous but also ever-shifting, evolving, and moving. We do not enter the now static—we enter it present in the moment-to-moment. We go with the reality; we do not get carried away or held back by thoughts.

In the garden, we acclimate plants, we amend soil, we graft, we train fruit trees, we apply frost protection, we make shade devices, and we bring plants inside for winter—we make modifications. Adaptation is part of the doings of a gardener. Everything is in flux; we are in flow with it. The rigid branch is lost in a storm; the pliant and adjusting gardener is ready for the challenges.

Challenge is good. Change is good. Mindfulness is subtly adjusting neural pathways to become more pliant and adaptive—mindfulness naturally supports neuroplasticity. Mindfulness adapts your mind, body, and spirit to encounter the moment-to-moment of your lived experience as a fuller, more fulfilling experience.

Successional Sowing

Gardeners know the trick of not sowing the whole packet at once but rather staggering it in smaller batches. A variety of maturities extends the season of that plant's interest or yield and creates a more robust garden. A March second sow is also a backup to any potentially frost-hit February sowings. It reminds us that resilience is not just an ability to bounce back but a matter of preparation too.

Mindfulness is not a "happy place" bubble to avoid reality or escape from life struggles. It is the successional sowing of intent and the repeated germination of awareness—it is entering reality and being equipped to not only be resilient but also take it all in stride.

This book may have you smell more than one rose or pull more than one weed. That's what we do in the natural world anyway, but it is also because repeat practice is the building of muscle memory. Repetition is the mastering and the reality of it.

The continual is the practice—make another drill.

Take a Moment to Feel the Warmth of the Sun

Sure, we may feel the sweat on our brow, but take a moment to feel the sensation of warmth. Notice and receive how the rays of the sun are felt on our skin. These are the rays that make our plants grow—drivers of transpiration and photosynthesis.

These are the rays that sustain the life of our garden. By acknowledging them for a moment, we may extend some appreciation or gratitude, but we are also in the moment of a more instant communication. We are sentient of their warmth directly—that is the language of the sun, and we instantly understand it. The sun shines that out. It is powerful in delivering that message.

By bringing our attention to the reality of how nature stimulates our sensations, we comprehend, and in receiving, we answer back. We shine our recognition, we signal our perception, and we are strong in our awareness—that's a powerful message.

The Nature of Thoughts

Thoughts are ideas, not directives. You don't have to follow every one to its conclusion. You don't even have to follow it a few steps. The whole point of mindfulness is to allow thoughts to arise but not cling to every one. The brain is in part a thinking machine—analyzing and making sense of the world around us and, on occasion, the emotional turbulence within us. It likes to busy itself with all that activity and excitement, but we don't have to play that game.

By all means, lasso the one that's going to set you free, make your fortune, or revolutionize society, but there is no need to ride out every bucking and panicking idea. We can be prompted into action by thoughts—that's their actual mechanism—but we can, being mindful, just let them be a transitory moment as well. Ideas can be good or bad—picked up or dropped.

Some ideas are viable, attractive seed; some are weeds. You don't have to cultivate every plant that sprouts in the garden. You get to choose.

"Within you, there is a stillness and a sanctuary to which you can retreat at any time and be yourself."

—Hermann Hesse

Weeding Preconceptions

If spontaneous thoughts are the annual weeds—the daily ask—then our preconceptions (or mindset attitudes) are the perennial weeds, the story constantly told. We can stop ourselves from grasping a thought, but it's harder not to grasp an attitude.

In the actual garden, we know that annual weeds can have their heads hoed off and decapitation is death, while perennial weeds may spring up two more shoots after a slice back and so need a deeper rooting out. It's not so different in the psychological realm. In the early days of mindfulness, you will easily tackle the annual-type thoughts—those that just pop up from time to time—but your deep-rooted, ingrained thinking patterns will take a little longer. The more you slice, the more you diminish the root's regeneration capacity, and eventually you will deplete it of all reserves and win this war of attrition.

The more mindful and consciously positive, open, and compassionate experiences—and intentions—that blossom in the garden of your being, the less room there is for perennial weeds. Over time, the root network of your thriving plants dominates the ground and yields no space for a weed to take root. An impermeable barrier of living goodness and resilient fortitude—this is the rewiring neuroplasticity of mindfulness. This is mindful gardening of the soul.

Go Get Your Hands Dirty

Doing brings the reward of achievement. Accomplishment is a trigger to positive endorphin release and a feel-good factor. While mindfulness is not about a high, it is about heightened experience; it is about higher purpose. In fuller health, we are more energized to really live. Getting your hands dirty in the garden is a true motivation for that.

We should acknowledge our gardening and life achievements more to tilt a positive bias. We gardeners too often move on to the next thing on the to-do list and don't fully allow the accomplishment to register. Mindfully register your good work today. Do that more often.

"I did well" and "that made a difference" are not dirty words—it is not ego at play; it is acceptance of a truth. You did do well; that did make a difference. Dirty your hands with some of that positive loam. Make a fine tilth for positive bias.

Handling Joy

The poet Alfred Austin (1835–1913) once noted, "The glory of gardening: hands in the dirt, head in the sun, heart with nature." It turns out that getting your hands dirty may have some health benefits. Yes, be conscious of the neighborhood cat's droppings or the sharp shards in your soil, but handling soil may be medicating you toward joy.

Soil is the life of the garden. Soil contains life—including bacteria known as *Mycobacterium vaccae*, which increase serotonin release in humans upon contact. We gardeners have regular contact with this soil microbe—we can inhale or ingest a little from particles blown up into breathable air, make topical contact with it and absorb it through our green fingers and soil-working hands, and get it directly in the bloodstream via any nick on our skin.

As we work the garden, this antidepressant particle works us—in the direction of clarity, confidence, and a greater sense of physical and mental well-being. Today in the garden, mindfully acknowledge the joy it brings you—in the doing, in the being, and in the interaction with life, including tiny, mind-altering bacteria.

Handling Anger

Theravada Buddhism teaches that the antidote to anger is compassion and loving-kindness. This is not the easiest of asks, but it's necessary when we accept that anger is toxic not just to the spirit but also to the body, which it floods with a stressful chemistry. In mindfulness, we learn to master our emotions—or at least not have them dominate us.

I admit that I am not quite at the stage of extending goodwill or loving-compassion to the slugs that devour my seedlings—although I want to be of Buddha mind and Krishna consciousness. I do, however, acknowledge that they are only operating within their nature—feeding and living; there is no malice. There is no need for a sense of injustice or anger. It is just the nature of the garden. It is just the nature of life—there are things beyond our control, and bad things happen; we cannot internalize everything that does not go according to plan or our peace of mind. We don't have to ride the storm or the tsunami of negative emotion; we can bring compassion to our self and move on to the next moment.

Anger, doubt, regret—all the disrupting sentiments— are just sentiments. They are not you; they are not of "I" or "mine." They are transitory, if you let them transit on—if you transition to a different now. Slugs eat. We garden. Life goes on.

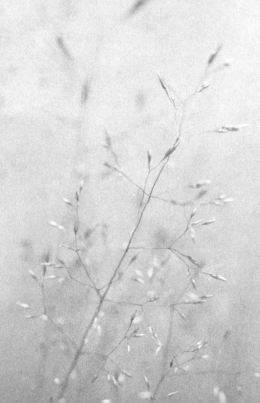

"The leaves of the tree are many but the root is one.
When the root is firm the branches flourish."

—Chinese proverb

Transmutation

Anger can be motivation. I know that to many practitioners and gurus on the spiritual path, ego and anger are seen as evils. I dispute that. It is the context. Perhaps egotism can go, but you can't obliterate the self fully. You still need some self for self-respect, self-esteem, self-reliance, and self-control.

The letting go is not of any semblance of self; rather, it is letting go of self-identification with aggression, greed, emotional pain, and other suffering. It is transcending the moment—that is going to heaven, that is reaching nirvana, and that is the journey and the afterlife or, should I say, the next stage of life.

Anger is problematic, but it often stems from what we perceive as an injustice. That hints at a will to right the situation, but we can stand in front of the tank, not drive it. We can lovebomb and not blow up. We can overcome. We can better channel the energy.

Anger is a human trait, so if it's good enough for evolution to retain, then it has some value. I do not mean aggression; I mean a sense of justice or outrage at injustice or true evils. Anger is the sensation we experience when something offends us. If the smirk of a colleague angers, work on that. If slavery, persecution, or prejudice offends you, then get to work on that—vote, campaign, boycott, and speak up.

So if those slugs are still bothering you into rage or clenched teeth, then be motivated by it—make the beer trap, buy the grit, and protect the plants. Turn the negative experience into an impetus for a more positive experience. This is the alchemy of the soul. There is more to make than precious metals.

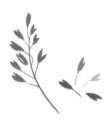

Growing with Compassion

Compassion is not just an emotional response to a situation; it is a human drive. It is part of what humans do. It might even be the answer to how we can be. Compassion doesn't have to be cosuffering; it can be loving expression. Compassion may be empathy or sympathy at first, but it is always good intention toward the transmutation of pain. And like all good alchemy, it transmutes our brain chemistry—with a flood of oxytocin, the bonding and well-being transmitter.

The more we experience or practice compassion, the more brain circuits that are receptive to this care and pleasure get strengthened. The more that our sympathetic and empathetic intelligence is expressed, the less that negative emotional links are fired. Compassion and forgiveness are shown to decrease feelings of anger, hatred, jealousy, depression, and self-doubt. Compassionate meditations decrease rumination, enhance communication skills, and strengthen our sense of human connection.

Physically, compassion slows heart rate, lowers stress hormones, increases immune function, strengthens the vagus nerve and cardiac circulation, and bolsters the pathways of alert presence. Compassion brings us to our true selves—alive and vibrating love.

Sowing Self–Compassion

Most of us are raised to be kind to others. Most of us find that not just in the home and schooling of our developmental years but also in the faith-system teachings that our parents, community, or culture introduces us to, there's a universal "be kind" law—be nice to others. Not always do we pick up the message or tenet of "be kind to yourself"—and therein a life of turbulence abounds.

On one level, self-compassion involves treating yourself the way you would treat anybody else who may be suffering or going through a hard time— with consideration, nonharshness, nonjudgment, and support. Self-compassion is not self-indulgence—it is not self-pity. It is breaking free of pity and rumination and accepting pain and suffering for what they are— transient. It is seeing and accepting the reality of your situation and not worsening it. It is letting it be—and pass without blame or shame.

We can mindfully observe our pain or current trouble and not add to it with self-criticism or reactionary thought. Self-compassion is addressing the wound, not picking at it or wishing it away. Self-compassion is being real with yourself. As we mindfully garden and mindfully live our lives, self-compassion becomes easier. As we befriend ourselves through mindfulness, it is easier to be friendlier to our self.

A body scan is a good way to check in with our physical self, but doing it with the intent of extending loving-kindness and positive energy into each part is a loving act toward the self. It is the compassionate hug that we might give to another person.

Allowing yourself to fully enjoy your gardening experience today is a gift to the self too. It is not a salve or a distraction; it is the way through—it is the connection to your true self even when hurt. It is accepting hurt and choosing to live.

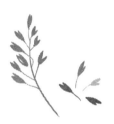

Gardening with the Seasons

Gardening is a year-round activity. We gardeners encounter nature in every month of the year and get to truly witness how the year unfolds, observing the rhythms and the specifics of each season. Nongardeners may observe the seasonal changes at some point—often through a window or via a change in wardrobe—but we get to bear witness and participate in the cyclical return of each stage of the year. We get to live with and through it—be fully present to the beauty and truth of it.

Not only is there awe and inspiration in each season, but by being in each season—present to each change and subtle shift—we can appreciate the true reality of the world. We can move more freely in every moment-to-moment of the year and become more in harmony with the natural world and our natural selves. As gardeners, we learn to accept and embrace change, we get resilient, and we get other rewards too.

If we are kitchen gardeners, we get to eat in season—real food of the moment, not out of sync or commercially forced food; this is the engine of health. Summer foods are packed with phytochemicals that help our bodies deal with environmental stresses; autumn foods have agents that ward off bacterial infection and help humans do likewise; winter foods have plenty of antiviral and antidepressant chemistry, just as we need both; and come spring, greens can break down any fats or toxins accumulated over winter. Being in sync is really good.

Being in and of the season is being in the correct now—in the right place, in the right manner, in receipt of nature's bounty and a more natural support of health and activity. There is abundance in being a mindful gardener, and there are abundant opportunities to flex some gratitude and some sheer fascination.

Where are you in the year now? Meet it, notice it, experience it, and live it.

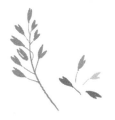

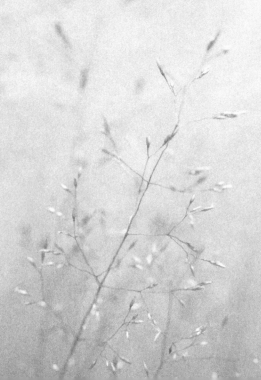

"To forget how to dig the earth and to tend the soil is to forget ourselves."

—Mahatma Gandhi

A Lie on the Grass

When did you last just lie down on your lawn and look up at the sky? A lie on the grass is not just a pleasant rest; it evokes the awe-inspired carefree activity of childhood—a transportation to a time long before embarrassment became a barrier to being happy-go-lucky.

Lying on the grass is a way to be earthed and grounded. That's true not just in the spiritual sense—where you let the earth take the weight of yourself and you release your tensions into it and realize your gratitude for being alive in this moment—but also in the process of detoxing any static buildup in your body that may be contributing to brain fog, inflammation, muscle tension, decreased immune function, and fatigue. Lying on the grass puts you in direct contact with the healing polarity of the magnetic field of the earth. It is more than the time-out that reenergizes.

Lie down—read a book, cloud-gaze, feel the warmth of the sun's rays, have your lunch break, or have a proper do-nothing time-out; just do it horizontally, in contact with the earth. You can allow appreciation or gratitude. You can consciously deepen your awareness of the moment—really acknowledge the experience. You can release your body tension into the holding arms of the earth. You can let go of thoughts—make it a mindful lie on the grass.

Giving Thanks

Every culture around the world has developed rituals and ceremonies conducted in springtime to give thanks for new growth. That's not just because the plants newly emerging around us are sustenance—new food, new medicine, new materials for clothing and shelter, and new dyes and material for decoration and creative expression—but also because spring heralds the renewal of the new.

New plants emerging signify the awe of the continual—of the regeneration of life; of course that rejuvenates the spirits. Why wouldn't we want to dance, sing, and share food? Why wouldn't we want to tie a ribbon to a tree, paint our bodies, or make a pilgrimage to a place of natural wonder? Every culture has evolved mechanisms to give thanks for the harvest come autumn. We bookend the growing season with joyful gratitude.

No matter which part of the year it is, today is a good day to give thanks to the garden we work and tend, which rewards with so much pleasure, promise, and positive regard for the natural world. Who needs a temple to pray in when you have a garden? And if I may paraphrase some divine liturgy, then yes, it is right to give thanks and praise. Certainly, it's more than a yes to a moment or two engaged in appreciative mindful meditation.

To Potter

Mindfulness and other spiritual and psychological techniques and practices are often framed in "being"—in being calm, in slowing down and focusing on your inner being, in allowing yourself to just "be": to be unburdened, to be well, and to be cured. But while being is great, if you cannot be, you must become—and that, for some, takes a little doing. Over the course of this book, we have been doing; after this book, we will keep doing.

The easiest doing in the garden is a potter-about—so why not take a lead from that and have a leisurely but conscious stroll around your garden? This easy mode is still a means to connect with nature and your true self. Just potter; as you go, inhale the power of the place and exhale your appreciation and gratitude for its gift and bounty. Move through it, and let it move you. Here is joy; here is home. Here is your awakened presence.

You don't have to be of singular purpose to achieve dynamic states of consciousness. The amble and the potter—the chill-out and relaxed participating—can be just as real. They can really deliver a moment of at-oneness with your surroundings and yourself.

With your being in your doing, there is nothing amiss.

Appreciating Rain

In addition to watering the garden and wild plants, rain washes leaves clean of dust and debris, which unblocks stomata (plant pores) and allows them to open and close more efficiently. Improving the gaseous exchange not only facilitates how a plant grows and reaches upward but also helps take pollutants out of breathing air and replenishes the planet with oxygen. Rain is life on so many levels.

The best time to do a rain dance is not before but during. Gratitude toward natural rhythms means being in rhythm with nature. So go on—shake a tail feather. Show a physical manifestation of a little positive regard. It is liberating to do so—overcome your embarrassment, and embrace a joyous pulse of life.

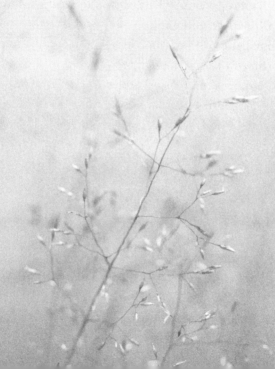

"*True happiness is to enjoy the present, without anxious dependence upon the future, not to amuse ourselves with either hopes or fears but to rest satisfied with what we have, which is sufficient, for he that is so wants nothing.*"

—Seneca

The Lesson of Autumn Leaves

Spring and summer leaves go about their business of photosynthesis. From the energy of the sun and elements in the air and soil, they manufacture the plant sugars that produce energy to grow and survive. In the lessening light of autumn, photosynthesis begins to slow and slow, and so for some plants, their leaves are no longer efficient machines or helpful additions. They are a drain on resources, or at least they add nothing. The plants pull the sugars and phytochemicals back into their stems and roots to conserve energy—to get through the winter and into the spring. Soon they will shed their foliage altogether and make new leaves in a more appropriate season.

Autumnal leaves are surplus to requirement, so trees let them go. The lesson we may take away is that it is good to be enriched, but it is also natural to let go.

A Latitude for Gratitude

Gardening gifts myriad opportunities to be grateful. Grateful that the sun is shining or that the wind has abated or that the rain is doing the watering today. Grateful that those seeds germinated or that plant flowered or that bush berried. We gardeners can mistake our kind regard for the situational moment as relief—relief that the sun is shining or the wind abated, etc. But by becoming more mindful, we shift our contentment to joy and lift our relief to thankfulness—to a deeper appreciation of the situation. To not just sense the happening of a good moment but also embrace and rejoice that the moment is good for you too.

Many studies have found that expressing or experiencing gratitude can trigger a realization of eudaemonia; that's a positive psychological perception of one's own welfare, often accompanied by a sense of physical health. Being thankful is so close to being joyful that our brain chemistry and body respond accordingly. Gratitude is now popular as a psychological device to protect oneself from stress, negativity, self-pity, anxiety, and depression. Long before that, it was simply a way to count your blessings.

Put the trowel down for a moment, and feel for that eudaemonia. Put the trowel down because, if you count the blessings of the garden, you will need both hands.

Cultivating Eudaemonia

Of course, you can pick up the trowel and cultivate some eudaemonia. The concept of eudaemonia is as old as the Greek gods, but it is perhaps most clearly considered in Aristotle's *Nicomachean Ethics*, where it is understood to mean "to live and fare well." Etymologically, it consists of the words *eu*, meaning "wellness," and *daimōn*, which denotes a guardian spirit. So it is the spirit of doing good—thriving.

It is often translated as welfare, well-being, happiness, flourishing, blessedness, prosperity, and so on. It's not a bad thing to be cultivating. So how do we grow this good life? Well, by growing things and enjoying them, by eating our harvest, by looking forward to our next sowing, and by participating in our pleasures and our rewarding pastimes.

Appreciating the garden and mindfully considering the more positive aspects of life is often seen as having a positive outlook. But it is a personality trait that can be honed more if you naturally have it—and gained if it's not your natural inclination. The way is to express more gratitude, kind regard, and loving-kindness toward yourself, your daily experiences, and your life journey.

It is not so difficult. It is just a matter of allowing it. Take the time to appreciate the beauty or bounty of the next plant you water. Take the time to notice the next pollinating bee. Bring your awareness to how good it is to be outside as your flourishing self in your flourishing garden.

The Old Joke

There is an old joke that it is hard to tell: Where does the garden start and the gardener end? There is truth in this, of course—great effort may be required to physically construct a garden and to maintain it in the realms of your projected perfection thereafter.

There is even a fridge magnet that says, "The garden is a thing of joy . . . and a job forever." But the spiritual truth in it is that we merge—the gardener and the garden are one. There is no taking apart or separating. In this merging, we find our true nature there. That's the last laugh.

"Close your eyes, fall in love, stay there."

—Rumi

Just Sit and Relax

It is time for a time-out. There's no need to follow your breath or fully switch on. Go have a do-nothing moment out in the garden—in your favorite spot. You can mind-wander—no bother. You can look around or just listen. Whatever—no matter; just sit and be in it.

It is not hard work to rest. It is not hard work to appreciate resting. It is okay not to strive. It is good to sit and relax and not try to become—to just be in whatever mood you are in, in whatever state manifests. Sit and be.

Be of no fuss at all. This, too, is a powerful prayer.

The Solace of Solitude

Gardening can be a solitary pastime, but it's rare we feel alone there. The garden is a comforting space, full of your creativity and your nurturing care. There are times when it wraps its arms back around you as you have done for it, but being a gardener also develops a resilient nature—we work it alone, we spend our time there often in silence and without any wows. In times of stress and pain, a step out into the garden refires that long-wired aspect—the solace button is pushed.

Many of the great mystics found solace in their silence and solitude—in the quiet alone, there is personal renewal. In the quiet alone, there is a deepening of the grace of self-strength—of bringing to the moment your capacity for unfretful stillness and spiritual grounding, of being here or there no matter what. That's not just a comfort; that's fortitude.

Gardening strengthens our capacity to be alone—that does not mean we become loners and removed from sociability. It means not desperate—never being alone for fear of loneliness or what you might begin to feel or think if left to your own devices. It is self-confidence. It is self-awareness. It is replenishing.

There is no fear of missing out when you are busy pruning a bush or planting a planter. There's no need to find out what's going on beyond—it is all here, all you need, all that needs you: the union of self and true nature. In the solitude of the garden, there is the escape from the noise of the constructed and confounding world. The quiet alone is music to many ears.

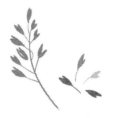

A Real Measure

Gardening brings us into the rhythms of the natural world. We experience the seasons in real time and the day's weather in real time—we are real in our time spent there.

Today, deepen your awareness of the moment of the year we are in right now. Notice the ambient temperature, the light levels, and the stage of growth or recession of the garden. It is unmissable what season we are in. You can look at an app or the kitchen calendar, but stepping into the now of nature is the real measure of reality. This moment is meeting nature and looking nature in the eye—this experience of the true reality of this moment is entering reality fully. This is "awake presence."

Notice the Everyday

Sometimes we want to be wowed or awestruck by something spectacular, and that's okay. But don't forget to notice the wow and awe in the everyday. When we notice, we break free of autopilot mode and find that our feet are our wings to soar.

As gardeners, we may find it all too easy to bring our presence to the task—we love it so much. It is easy to be attentive to watering, weeding, or planting because when we garden we connect with life, and when we connect with life we come alive.

When you come alive waiting for a bus or drinking coffee or getting dressed in the morning, that's when you have really come into life. All those garden chores mindfully carried out are strengthening neural pathways that make it easier to transition from mindful gardener to everyday mindfulness—to be your authentic and attentive self in the rest of your life.

"Flow with whatever may happen, and let your mind be free: Stay centered by accepting whatever you are doing. This is the ultimate."

—Zhuang Zhou

Keep Doing What You Love

The more you do what you love, the more love you bring into the world. Cherish every seed and flower. Appreciate every gardening day and every season for their own rewards and actions. Enjoy yourself and your *self* as your most inspired, in flow, beautiful self.

Cultivating the garden is more than cultivating plants; it is cultivating ourselves. It is the opening of verdant hearts; it is the birthing of love. Aphrodite may have emerged from an ocean, but the first thing she did was pick a rose.

Keep cultivating with love. Keep cultivating love.

Getting Lost and Found in the Garden

This book started with an observation on getting lost in the garden. The "lost in the garden" experience is what psychotherapists, sports psychologists, and counselors might describe as finding your flow. It is being completely absorbed in an activity but fully there, present to it, with your full potential in it. You are not really lost in it; you are found in it.

Mindful practitioners would suggest that the final step to attaining total mindfulness is the one in which you find your "flow." Working in the garden, systematically watering or weeding without distraction and focused on the task, is one of the surest and shortest routes to your flow—to a natural, sustained mindfulness.

Getting lost in the garden is a valid way of finding mindfulness, peace of mind, awe, peak experience, and awareness. Getting lost in the garden is a way to let your true self be found.

Acknowledgments

I am a believer that all creativity is a conversation. There is always a bigger picture with multiple contributors, and certainly there are people who have influenced my spirit as much as the spirit of this book—the likes of Anthony de Mello, Thich Nhat Hanh, and Lao Tzu. Some are quoted in these pages, and some are featured in the bibliography. There are also those family, loved ones, and friends who keep a lookout when I am engrossed in the realms of thought and writing and make sure that I am watered, fed, and well weeded. And then there are those who have nurtured the book in hand and kept it watered, fed, and well weeded, so a special thanks to Fiona Hallowell, Michael Croland, and all the team at Dover/Ixia for their support and encouragement.

Bibliography

Analayo, Bhikkhu. *Satipatthana: The Direct Path to Realization*. Birmingham, UK: Windhorse Publications, 2004.

Baer, Ruth A. *Mindfulness-Based Treatment Approaches: Clinician's Guide to Evidence Base and Applications*. Burlington, MA: Academic Press, 2006.

Cleary, Thomas. *Practical Taoism*. Boston: Shambhala, 1996.

Hanh, Thich Nhat. *Interbeing: Precepts for Everyday Living*. Berkeley: Parallax Press, 1987.

Hanson, Rick, and Richard Mendius. *Buddha's Brain: The Practical Neuroscience of Happiness, Love and Wisdom*. Oakland: New Harbinger Publications, 2009.

Kabat-Zinn, Jon. *Wherever You Go, There You Are: Mindfulness Meditation in Everyday Life*. New York: Hyperion Books, 1994.

Kornfield, Jack. *The Wise Heart: A Guide to the Universal Teachings of Buddhist Psychology*. New York: Bantam, 2008.

Siegel, Daniel J. *Aware: The Science and Practice of Presence— The Groundbreaking Meditation Practice*. New York: TarcherPerigree, 2018.

Silananda, Sayadaw U. *The Four Foundations of Mindfulness*. Somerville, MA: Wisdom Publications, 1990.

Tanahashi, Kazuaki. *The Heart Sutra: A Comprehensive Guide to the Classic of Mahayana Buddhism*. Boston: Shambhala, 2016.

About the Author

Fiann Ó Nualláin is a lifelong gardener, by passion and profession. His horticultural vocation has seen him move from plant cultivation and medicinal botany to award-winning garden design. He has taught continuing education horticulture classes and developed social and therapeutic horticulture projects with schools, health care facilities, state agencies, and local communities.

Fiann writes a weekly gardening column for the *Irish Examiner* and regularly contributes gardening advice and well-being slots on Irish national television and radio. Fiann is the author of several books on practical herbalism, including the best-selling *Natural Cures for Common Ailments* and *Beauty Treatments from the Garden*. He is also the author of *By Time Is Everything Revealed*, published by Ixia Press, an exploration of mindfulness and life wisdom contained in Irish proverbs.